2020

Connections

TODD WEBER, PHD

Connections:
Aging, Crossfit, Community, and Quality of Life

Copyright @ 2020 Todd Weber
All Rights Reserved

June 2020

Crossfit plays a big part in this book and it is important to note that I am talking about Crossfit at the affiliate level, not the corporate level. Recently Crossfit at the corporate level had quite a shake-up.

Greg Glassman, the former owner and CEO of Crossfit, made comments about Black Lives Matter and the recent killings of black males by police that were considered racist and very inappropriate. As a result, many affiliates and Crossfit athletes protested and withdrew from being a part of Crossfit. Crossfit Oregon City was one box that chose to drop affiliation.

Greg Glassman stepped down as CEO but remained as owner of Crossfit. That did not satisfy many people and the pressure was on Crossfit to make sweeping changes.

An affiliate owner from Colorado stepped forward and bought Crossfit from Glassman. He made all the right moves in taking ownership and promises many changes. Only time will tell if that happens.

CFOC, like many affiliates, remains on hold to see how it plays out. CFOC stands firmly in solidarity with Black Lives Matter. If that had not been the case, many of us would have changed boxes to one that did.

Contents

Chapter One

Chapter Two

Chapter Three

Chapter Four

Chapter Five

Chapter Six

Chapter Seven

Chapter Eight

Chapter Nine

Chapter Ten

Chapter Eleven

Chapter Twelve

Chapter Thirteen

Chapter Fourteen

Chapter Fifteen

Chapter Sixteen

Introduction

In this book I hope to show connections between many disparate areas of our lives that impact our health and fitness as older or aging athletes. By athletes, I mean anyone who is or wants to be active, healthy and fit – starting at any point in the fitness spectrum. You may not have worked out for decades. You may be chronically ill. You may be so overweight that it is hard to get off the couch. Or you may be in good shape and ready for new challenges. It doesn't matter what your age or gender is… although this book is aimed more for the older athlete.

And by health, I mean not just our bodies, but our minds, spirit, and capacity to contribute to issues larger than ourselves.

We live in times that are full of differences. There are extreme political views. Our environment is under full attack from climate change and pollution. Our social structures are changing rapidly. There are so many versions of the "truth" that it is hard to pick solid ground.

My generation, the "Boomers", were going to change the world. We were going to stop wars. We were going to create the Age of Aquarius. We challenged the "Establishment" on every front. Human rights, equal rights for women, civil rights, and more were all targets for change.

We managed to force a President out of office and make strides in many areas. Then we got co-opted by mortgages, 2-car garages, both spouses working, and prosperity. We became semi-dormant for decades. And for many of us, we became complacent. And we got old.

But old isn't what it used to be! 70 is the new Black and longevity is much different now. We are at a place in our lives where we have time and resources. The world needs our passion, knowledge, and strength to address the issues that are at the tipping point. We need to re-join the fight and we need to be strong and fit to do it.

Please join me in getting fitter, stronger, and healthier. We need to be able to step forward to create healthier communities, a healthier environment, and healthier mindsets. Our children, grandchildren and great-grandchildren need our help if we are going make changes big enough to avoid the tipping points.

Connections
Crossfit, Aging, and Wholeness

I am turning 70 years old this week. I am a typical American male who spent 40 years behind a desk. I had all the signs of wear and tear to show for it…slumped, rounded shoulders, head thrust forward, shuffling walk. I had aches and pains from imbalances and old injuries and poor nutrition. I was fairly sure I was "over the hill" and things would only get worse. Then an amazing thing happened 20 months ago. I started aging backwards.

No, really! At seventy years old, my resting heart rate is 42. My sleeping respiration is 15. My body scan done last week shows that in the last six weeks I gained 4.2 pounds of lean muscle mass, lost 4.4% body fat, and gained just over half an inch in height. The height difference happened over the course of a year and one-half. This is all a continuation of positive changes that started 20 months ago when I found Crossfit.

According to the healthcare industry and the fitness industry and big Pharma and the internet weight-loss/fitness gurus and the other vested interests who want to perpetuate the current myths on aging, this should not be possible. Or, if it does happen, it is because of hormone treatments and steroids. I assure you that this is not about hormones or steroids.

I am writing this book to share the insights and information that I've gained over 40 plus years of interdisciplinary study. That, and being an on-again off-again athlete since I was a child. Joining crossfit 20 months ago started the process of making connections linking all my studies and readings with the amazing changes happening to my body.

I am not doing this because I want to sell you a new fitness plan or weight-loss system. I don't want to sell you anything. In fact, I want you to question and doubt everything I have to say in this book and not take it as true until you have tested it against your own experience and value systems. As the Buddha said, Question everything.

This book is written after 40 years of exploring and learning and questioning many different things. It is about the connections I've made (or others made) between many disparate areas: science, spirituality, fitness, health, psychology, intention, community, social construction, and many more topics.

I invite you to enjoy the ride. Be skeptical. Be a student. Be a beginner. I hope to pull it all together by the end of the book. Then you can let me know what you think.

I will provide references at the end of the book. A lot of what is presented does not have a direct or clear path to previous authors' works or I read it and digested it so many years ago that I can't remember where it came from. Just assume none of this material is new, that I gleaned it from others, and they deserve the credit for the ideas. I simply am the messenger trying to pull it together.

Thanks.

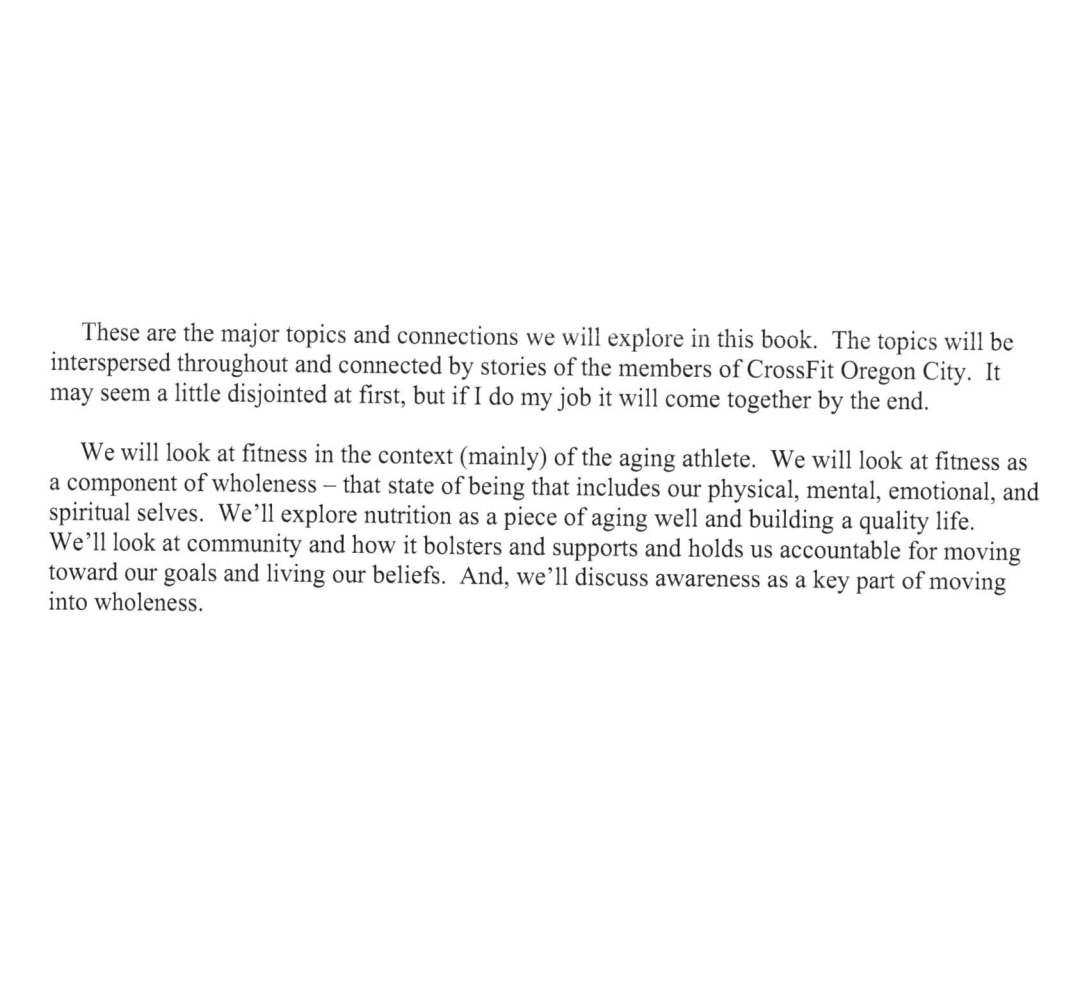

These are the major topics and connections we will explore in this book. The topics will be interspersed throughout and connected by stories of the members of CrossFit Oregon City. It may seem a little disjointed at first, but if I do my job it will come together by the end.

We will look at fitness in the context (mainly) of the aging athlete. We will look at fitness as a component of wholeness – that state of being that includes our physical, mental, emotional, and spiritual selves. We'll explore nutrition as a piece of aging well and building a quality life. We'll look at community and how it bolsters and supports and holds us accountable for moving toward our goals and living our beliefs. And, we'll discuss awareness as a key part of moving into wholeness.

Chapter One

It was the best of times; it was the worst of times...
Charles Dickens

We live in challenging times. Bad news is instantly available through the internet and TV. The slant on the news is to give bad news priority – disasters, accidents, wars, clashes, shootings, bombings, catastrophizes – and to paint as bleak a picture as possible.

Our culture is addicted to the negative. We can spot problems in a heartbeat and rarely, if ever, look for the positive. We are subjected to conflict all day – in politics, religion, economy, education, climate, healthcare and more. Of course, it feels like the worst of times.

Coexisting with that is the best of times. We have unimaginable technological capability. We have made huge strides in medicine, transportation, communication with many more breakthroughs just around the corner.

Yet, anxiety and stress are almost unbearable for many people.

The places we used to go for relief from this kind of pressure are no longer safe. We don't trust our government and politicians. Religion has become radicalized and political. Differences are magnified and used to divide us. It is a time when there are no clear solutions and truly little effort made to find common ground.

Our leaders have urged us to find ways of joining together to "Make America Great Again" and to become "A Thousand Points of Light." Yet we seemed to be more divided than ever.

In addition, we have an aging population that is riddled with lifestyle and metabolic diseases. We have a predetermined script for aging that includes words like "diminished," "weak," "vulnerable," "incapacitated," "senile," and many, many more.

The script goes something like this: As we age, we lose strength and bone density. We become more susceptible to diseases like cancer, diabetes, hypertension, obesity, dementia and many more. We need to be careful in case we "fall and can't get up." This script says aging is inevitable and there is nothing we can do about it, so we stop living and become "old."

Does this sound familiar? What if I say that this script is a load of crap? I believe we have bought into the script because it is delivered every day by the health care industry, big pharma, the food industry and many other "authorities" who gain big profits from this belief system.

This book explores connections where there might be a beginning to a different way of viewing what is happening. And it offers a much different approach than swallowing the old scripts whole and living much differently than we might have thought possible previously.

CrossFit is an organization that is about improving health and fitness. That may seem like a strange place to look for answers to these larger questions. However, in building and improving health and fitness, many other capacities are built and improved as well.

One of the major strengths of CrossFit is the communities that grow in every box. People who come together with a common goal to get fitter, stronger, healthier end up creating strong bonds and connections that are more than just an affinity for fitness. It also offers an alternative script and means to aging.

This book explores the experiences of members in one Cross Fit box in terms of the community and how the bonds and relationships create a place to change. The community comes together to do more than exercise. It gives back to the larger community in many ways. It creates hope. It creates action. And it creates love.

This is the story of health in the larger context of the term. It is the story of connections that become primary in peoples' lives. It is the story of people who care about themselves, about each other, and about the condition of their home, however that may be defined. It is a story of wholeness.

We will look at every aspect of crossfit at the local affiliate level and at the organizational level in terms of how it impacts members' experiences. We will focus mainly on the opportunities that Crossfit offers for aging differently. We will look at workouts, underlying principles, criticisms of cross fit, activities, and how the connections and bonds are created and grow.

The four main areas of focus in this book are exercise, nutrition, awareness, and community…and the connections to the larger aspects of life.

It is the start of a blueprint to change how we think about aging. It is a call to action to age differently. And it is an effort on my part to contribute a positive change to our world.

Fitness and health and all the related aspects are about quality of life. It is about the capacity to live fully into the later stages of life without being incapacitated by ill-health, poor strength and balance, and the inability to take care of ourselves.

In the larger scheme of things, this book is about aging athletes re-asserting their leadership in helping our country make changes to help get on track with our values and ideals. We are not a people or country who want to forcefully tear children away from their parents. We do not want to put people in detention camps depriving them of any rights and treating them inhumanely. We want to show leadership to the world in terms of a healthy and active democracy. We need to create an atmosphere of civil and respectful discourse – rather than lies and bullying and hate.

Crossfit boxes offer a model for communities that are safe, welcoming, health and fitness oriented, inclusive, and non-judgmental. We can all use a place like that in today's world.

In June 2017 I went to Kona Hawaii for a friend's wedding. At the time, I thought I was in reasonable shape for an older – but not elderly – man. I played golf a couple of times a week, ran occasionally and worked out with weights fairly often, but not consistently. Compared to other men my age I thought I must be in the top 10% in terms of physical shape. I weighed 275 pounds and was, I thought, 6'4".

Arriving at Kona, I saw several strange containers being offloaded from the plane with the baggage. It turned out that the containers held bicycles for athletes coming to Kona to compete in the age-group Ironman Triathlon. When traveling around the island that week I saw lean, fit athletes of every age.

My friend's wedding was great. We got to play golf a couple of times and then it was time to leave. At the airport while we waited to board the plane, I was watching many of the athletes who were also on the plane. It suddenly struck me that they were probably thinking about me the way I had thought many times about others: "I hope I don't have to sit next to that big dude!" I realized that I was the huge guy. I was not slim and fit as I once had been. And any chance I had of regaining fitness was past or slipping by quickly.

I turned to my friend and out of nowhere said, "I am going to lose 50 pounds by the end of September. I need you to hold me accountable." He looked at me and said that he couldn't hold me accountable, but he would help me keep track. I said that was good enough.

When I got home, I planned out how I was going to change my eating habits, I ran every day, and I looked for a Crossfit gym. I read about Crossfit and thought it might be the only fitness process that would work for me. If I went back to a typical commercial gym, I would just end up getting bored and quitting after a few months.

I looked at Yelp reviews for local Crossfit Boxes and found one that had wonderful reviews close by. I met with the owner the following week. And this is what happened:

Chapter Two

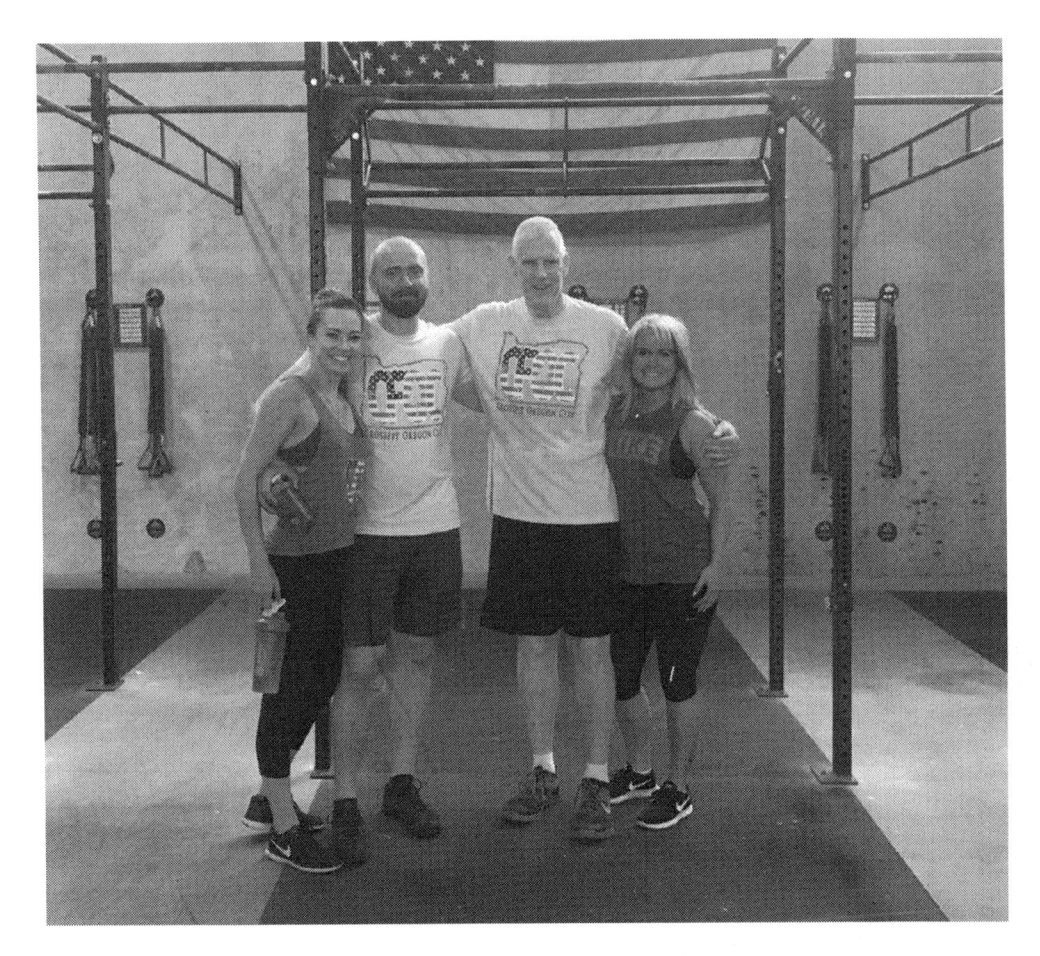

Cross Fit Oregon City (CFOC) is just like many other crossfit boxes. And, it is not. A box, by the way, is the term crossfit uses for a gym. CFOC has a robust, lively, healthy, welcoming, accepting, and supporting community that is unique in my experience – although common to the Crossfit organization. It is an amazing experience to be a part of.

One of the major themes I want to capture and share in this book is the essence of this community – the "special sauce" that is so meaningful to CFOC's members. We will also be exploring the fitness aspects – workouts, philosophy, and purpose. We'll take a hard look at nutrition and discuss the importance of sleep in a fitness routine. We'll talk about how our bodies hold tension and stress. We'll look at muscle imbalances and how they impact our quality of life. And, we will relate it all to aging.

The book is held together by the stories and experiences of the CFOC community as told to me by over 35 members through a series of interviews.

The members and owners of CFOC are amazingly open and giving in sharing their stories. Every interview moved me deeply and made me realize how lucky I am to be part of this.

Like you, I have a been a part of many groups and communities throughout my life. Groups and small communities make up the fabric of our culture. It is how we gain a sense of belonging to a place and time. It is how we connect with others to meet our social needs and desires. It is how we meet like-minded people to explore religion, politics, raising children, doing yoga, solving neighborhood issues, learning French, studying the bible, and much more. It is where we meet the significant people in our lives. It is where we make friends.

I found shelter with a group I didn't know existed. I found myself, at 68 years old, slipping closer and closer to being the person I promised I would never become. I was overweight and out of shape and it was getting harder to do activities that I once took for granted. I read about crossfit in men's fitness magazines and decided to give it a try. Being a lifetime member in commercial gyms – on and off – I knew I would not get what I needed by buying a new membership and giving up two months later. I needed a different approach.

I went online looking for crossfit gyms. There were several, so I looked at reviews and one box close to me stood out. That is how I found Cross Fit Oregon City.

I made an appointment to meet with one of the owners and my journey began. Here is some of what I found: hard exercise, weights, welcoming people, great coaching (like I have never had before), encouragement, support, celebration, suffering, connection, awareness of how truly unfit I was, acceptance, safety, cleanliness, passion, diversity, loud music, sweat (lots and lots of sweat), smiles and laughter (lots and lots of smiles and laughter), mental discipline, physical discipline, emotional support and growth, spiritual centeredness, and family. I found a family.

At the center of the CFOC experience are the two owners: Jen Cole Cereghino and Scott Cereghino. They set an extraordinary example. They give without measure. They support and encourage and coach and guide and when needed provide a shoulder to cry on or a cheer to celebrate. Every member of the box I interviewed talked about the impact Jen and Scott have on their lives. The other coaches are reflections of Jen and Scott. In different ways, they each give and share and support and goad and correct and push and slow down and envelope the athletes with love.

The community reflects all that. It brings tears to my eyes every time I think about it. It is so much fun. It is so warm and welcoming. It is so safe and accepting. It is so encouraging and supportive. It is so sweaty!

I hope you gain a view into this community and into crossfit. All the criticism of crossfit (and there is a lot of it out there) is mainly from competitors and vested interests with agendas. It does not seem to come from people who have experienced being in a box like CFOC.

Jen Cole Cereghino July 1st

Dr. Todd asked me a few weeks back what my MOST MEMORABLE moment/experience had been at CFOC- I, like many of you, have so many it's hard to list just one. But, this weekend's 24HEROESIN24HOURS stands out as one of my all-time most memorable for many reasons...

This weekend wasn't about a prize/award, it wasn't about who could lift the most, or who could complete the work the fastest, it wasn't a contest and there was no tangible "reward" for participating. We came together to honor those who could no longer do so, to bring awareness to a cause ([Navy SEAL Foundation](#)) which supports the spouses and children left behind... and, in doing so we all got to experience the power of community through the simple act of working out.

Thank you to those of you who committed your time to these workouts, even if it meant sacrificing sleep in doing so. Thank you to those who stuck around to keep us company and especially to those who jumped in on a workout because someone needed a teammate. Thank you to Beth for providing home-cooked meals throughout the night to share with anyone and everyone who wanted to partake. Thank you to Dr Kyle for providing recovery services in between your own workouts.

For me, this weekend epitomized our saying "Just Show Up"- many of you showed up not knowing the workout, showed up not knowing who you'd workout with, and/or not really knowing what to expect- and, because you did so, you met new people, worked out with someone you may not have worked out with, and exemplified the importance and impact of community. Thank you for always showing up and continuing to impress upon me and others the true meaning of friendship and camaraderie- it is experiences like this one which remind me why I fell in love with this "sport".

If you would like to CONTRIBUTE/DONATE to the Navy SEAL Foundation, for which this event was created, you may do so here:
https://www.crowdrise.com/o/en/campaign/cfoc/jencereghino

Saturday Morning Workout (WOD -Workout of the Day)

This workout is in preparation for a competition at the end of August. Many members of CFOC will be competing and/or supporting the competitors. As one of the members told me, CFOC travels well. We will have 100 members cheering for approximately 14 to 18 competitors. The competition is in Bend OR, across the Cascades into Eastern Oregon. I will be cheering.

The WOD looks tough. It is a partner WOD and I am expecting to do it with my mentee and friend Jason. I warm up and get my barbell, box, band for the pullups, and rower set up. The box is crowded from the early group who came to do a Tabata workout or to do the WOD earlier or who are working on special programming. The 9 o'clock group is huge – maybe 45 or 50 folks- which it tends to be on Saturdays. I am not worried that I don't see Jason yet. He is 17 and lives in a different reality than I, so I am not sure when he might be showing up.

At 9 o'clock Scott calls the group together to go over the workout – weights, movements, form- and asks if there are any questions. Then he asks if anyone needs a partner. I do not answer as I am still expecting Jason.

We warm up, do the movements with lighter weights to get the feel for the workout and are ready to start. No Jason. Close to me are two of the young beasts of the box – Tyler and Tyler. Both are in their mid-to-late twenties (I think) and can move mountains of weight and do every movement incredibly well. Before I could change my mind, I ask if I can shadow them for the workout. "Shadowing" is where a third person joins partners for a workout by working in rhythm with one of the partners. When that partner works, the shadow works, when that partner rests the shadow rests. My reps will not count toward the partner total. I will work to complete half the total reps set for the workout. I know I am about to get my butt kicked. And at the same time, I'm kind of excited that I get to work out with the "big boys."

The first 15-minute segment is a 150-calorie row. When that is complete, a 1 rep maximum thruster is established in the remaining time. I am a good rower and I feel super when I keep up and leave the rower at the same time as the team. Then I establish a new PR for a thruster and in the process, a new PR for a clean. I am totally pumped!

When the 15 minutes are up, Scott says "10 seconds" for the next phase. The next part of the workout is 100 alternating dumbbell snatches, 100 burpees to box jump, and 100 pullups. When doing the pullups, after each partner does a maximum effort, if the count is not 100, they must run 400 meters. Then keep going until 100 are completed...with a run after each partner's max effort if they are not at 100 yet. There is no time limit for completion. My part as the shadow is to do half the total for each movement and try to mirror the partner as much as possible.

I hold my own doing the DB snatches. I use a 20# dumbbell compared to the 50# dumbbell the Tyler's are using. It is called 'scaling" when an athlete changes the weight or movement to accommodate an injury or to make the workout as intense as it is designed to be without inviting an injury. In my case, it is plenty intense

50 snatches down and it is on to the burpees to box jump. Tyler and Tyler will be jumping to a 24" inch box. I am attempting to jump to a 12" box. They don't know it, but they have inspired me to jump to the box for the first time. Up until this point, I have been doing step ups. Seeing how these two athletes move gives me the confidence to try it. My form was not great, and I am sure that I forgot to do the burpee first about 1/3 of the time because I was concentrating on the jump, but it was so cool! I finish my 50 and they have waited for me to start the next movement!

50 pullups. Not my best movement. I use a band to help give support during the movement. I also have two max effort tries, as a master, before having to run 400 meters. I get 8 and 4 on my first two tries. T&T (we are getting closer now) do 15 and 20 their first tries. Remember we are doing these movements in a fatigued state after some very intense work. I am amazed at how many pullups they do. We run.

I get 5 and 3 this try. They continue to do an unbelievable number. They take off for the run, I do 400 meters on the rower.

I do another 8. They complete their 100. I row another 400 meters. I do another 8. My total is now 36. I am wiped out and wondering how I am going to finish. T&T and few other people come over and start cheering me. They tell me I can do it and give me advice to concentrate on one muscle group and then another and then another. I row 400 meters. I do another 8 – an extremely hard 8. I row 400 meters. I'm shaking and wondering how I will ever finish the final 6 reps. The crowd is cheering and supporting. I do not want to disappoint them. I do 4 reps. I am gasping for breath, feeling dizzy, but I only have 2 more to do. I jump up and get one rep and then an agonizingly slow 2nd one! I can't tell you how happy that made me. The "crowd" was 4 or 6 people. And they made me feel so loved. I pushed beyond limits I never thought possible and it was because some really good athletes let me workout with them and they helped me push past what I thought possible. That is crossfit.

    For an older athlete, getting to work with younger, fitter athletes is a blessing … and it is time to be careful. The younger athletes will push you in a way that you might not recognize and the unconscious need to compete creeps in. On the other hand, it is a good way to test your intensity and stamina. The main thing is to scale the workout so that it pushes you but does not put you in the path of an injury. Maturity plays a role here.
    I've found that the younger athletes like working out with me. I try to give it my best and they appreciate the effort I put out. After many workouts I've had younger members say to me that I helped push them and that they hope when they are my age, they will be pushing it that hard too.

Chapter Three

Brad Bremer 48 yrs old Firefighter CFOC since about 6 months after it started

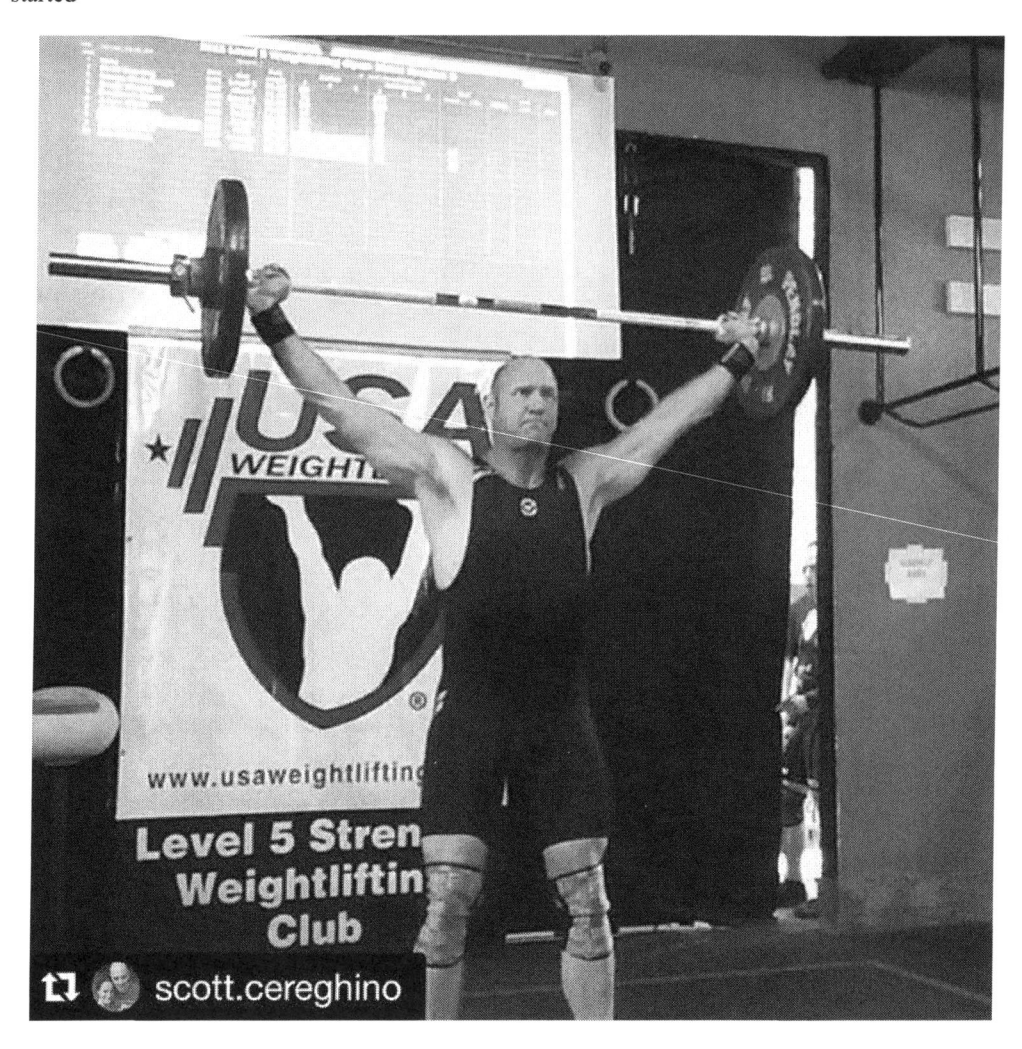

Brad is a big man with a big personality. He played high school football and spent 5 years in the army. He has always liked weights. As a firefighter/EMT, fitness is part of his job and he takes that seriously. He spent 10 years as a trainer at 24 Hour Fitness before discovering crossfit. He spent 6 months at a box where many of the firefighters at his station worked out. He saw the sign for CFOC, which is closer to his home, and decided to switch.

CFOC was small then – maybe 25 members- and Jen had a class for all new members before they could join regular classes. Brad met Jen one-on-one as he was the only new member right then. Brad gave her a little of his background and she asked him to do a few lifts – some squats and some cleans. He looked to her for a comment and she said, "It looks like we have some work to do."

Here is a guy who has been lifting weights for over ten years, is a personal trainer at a national gym system, and the last thing he expected to hear was there was work to do. Brad was laughing when he told me this story. He said, "She was right." She gave him a few corrections and he could feel the improvement immediately. Brad told me he was hooked!

He went on to become a coach at CFOC after obtaining his Level 1 certification from CrossFit. He also became a nationally ranked master's level Olympic Lifter, a certified masters level coach at the Colorado Springs Olympic Training Center, and a judge and official for Olympic lifting meets at every level.

Brad loves to coach. His passion and enthusiasm are contagious. He loves to work with people new to crossfit – to see them progress and accomplish their first push up or pull up! When he is telling me this he jumps up and pumps his fist. "We need to celebrate that!" he says. He explains that crossfit is not the Crossfit Games. We can do those workouts here – modified and scaled. But for Brad, it is about starting folks where they are and making each workout appropriate for their fitness level. Not easy – he grins – but appropriate. You need to listen to your body and make each workout what it is supposed to be in terms of intensity, duration, load, and so on. All the time he is talking he is getting louder and happier. He loves this stuff.

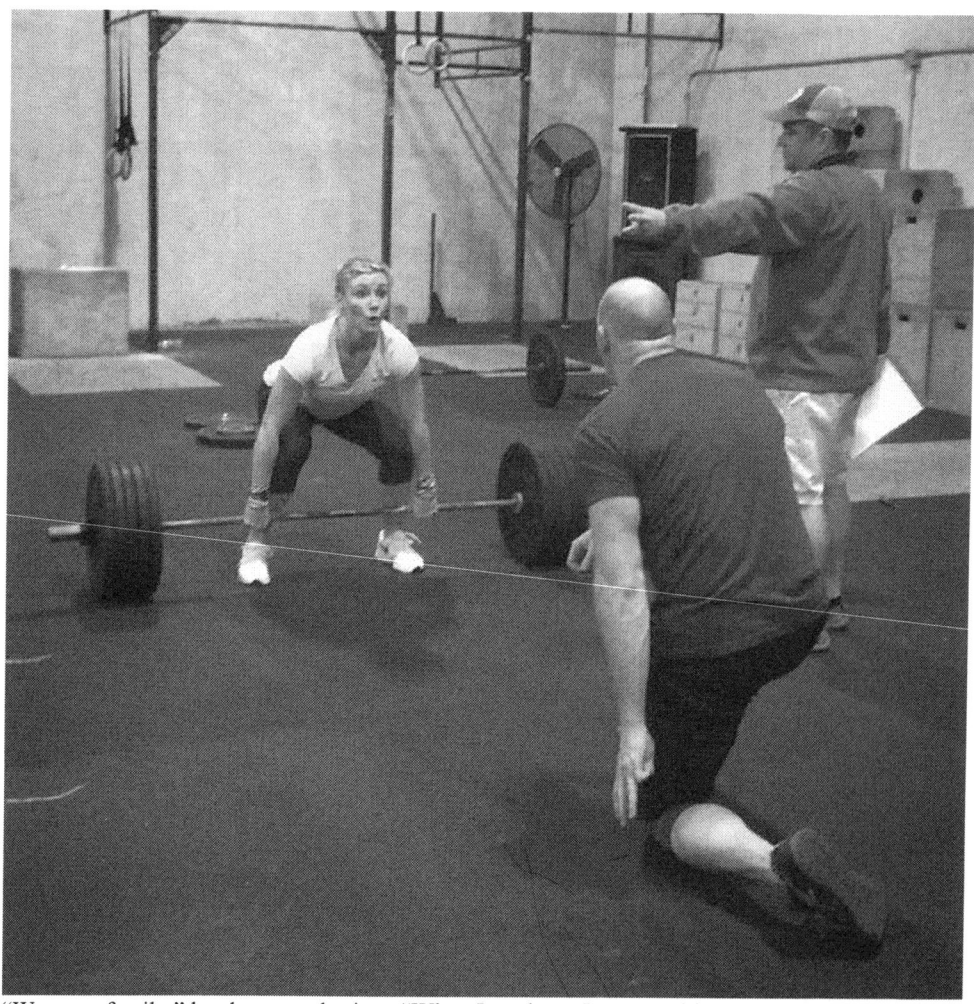

"We are a family," he shouts and grins. "When I am here, I am an athlete or a coach. I am part of the team. We support and encourage each other. We go through the suck together. And we come out closer on the other side."

"Jen is the special sauce," he says. She and Scott care. They set the example. She is the lifeblood of the box. She always takes the time to help.

He says that Jen has built a community on respect and admiration. It is not exclusive. Any one at any time can work out with any other person and feel secure and welcome.

Brad says that Jen wants every single member to feel confident and to feel included!

I must admit I was a little put off by Brad when I started at CFOC. I am a bit reserved and cautious until I get to know people and Brad is anything but reserved and cautious. About six weeks in, I was doing some work in the box on a Thursday. Thursday is skills day, meaning there is no regular WOD scheduled. People can make up a WOD that they missed or do a workout that is laid out or work on specific skills. There is no regular class. I use Thursdays as a recovery day and to work on skills that I need to improve or want to learn…which is all of them ⏵ I learned that I have a major muscle imbalance – my left side from the waist down (actually, it turns out, the whole left side) is much weaker than my right. I started physical therapy to work on it and they gave me several exercises to use to strengthen my weak areas.

I was working on those exercises and Brad came up to talk with me. I told him what I was doing, and he nodded saying that almost everyone has muscle imbalances and that he dealt with the same issue as me. He then showed me a stretch with a band that he used to warm up with that loosens the left side and makes it easier to move freely. It was really cool and worked well!

Then he went on to ask me what my goals were for crossfit. By now, it had become apparent to me that I was not the athlete that my wonky self-image thought I was and that I needed lots of help to just get the basics right. I was 68 years old then and still thought I was forty from the inside.

I told him this and he laughed and said, "Let's talk." He spent the next 20 minutes or so, without me asking, talking with me about mobility, movement, strength, and balance. Then he helped me outline a few realistic goals to reach by the first of the year. He said to me, "Todd, everyone comes in here and wants to be a Crossfit Games athlete overnight. Then they get realistic after a few workouts and understand that it is a long process and most of us will never be games athletes. So, they choose to focus on looking better, feeling better, and moving better. Then they start to get more fit and want to improve or gain a skill and they will ask for help during a workout – when we have limited time to give them the help they need." He went on to explain that during a workout he can offer tips for improving right then but can't address major mechanics or form or mobility issues.

He said to come in early or stay after class or to come in on Thursdays to work on the movements. It is the consistency that makes the difference. It doesn't happen overnight. Little by little the body adapts and creates a new way of moving. He said to me if I was consistent, I would make amazing progress.

I was so moved by his honest, open caring for me and that I could and would make progress if I chose to. He won me over right then. And, ever since he has helped me any chance he gets and always approaches me when he is there on Thursdays to see how I am doing and what I am working on. I can't express how important he is to me and how much I appreciate his help.

There is a lot of criticism of CrossFit by other elements of the fitness industry. One of the major points that is brought up often is how poorly trained Cross Fit affiliate coaches are and how dangerous the sport is because of that. Brad and the other coaches at CFOC show how wrong that criticism is.

I have been in and out of gyms for the past 50 years. I can tell you without hesitation that I have never been coached this well. I have never received such good personal feedback when I am working out. And I have never been shown this much concern about exercising safely.

In my experience, most of the big commercial gyms are more concerned with selling personal training than they are with good mechanics, form and safety.

I made more progress in two plus years at CFOC than I ever thought possible. Have I been sore? Oh yes! Has it been hard? You bet! And, that is part of the joy and celebration of getting fitter – everyday a little bit more.

I lost 55 pounds in the first 6 months. My body composition continues to improve with less body fat and more lean muscle mass. I move better than I have in decades. My posture is remarkably better. I am stronger and able to perform skills and movements I never thought would be possible at my age.

Is crossfit for everyone? Probably not. It is for anyone who wants to get fitter – yes, no matter what level and what age they are starting from. I am amazed at the changes I've made, and it just keeps getting better.

So, you ask, **why Crossfit** and not some other form of fitness for the older person? I am glad you asked!

Recent research in aging, evolutionary biology, and exercise physiology shows that "intense" physical exercise for 40 minutes a day or more turns on all kinds of mechanisms that fight aging.

The story, up until a few years ago, was that muscle and bone would wither and inevitably get weaker as we aged. Beginning around age 25 a person would a lose a percentage of strength every decade until in old age one would be a shriveled bag of bones. The only possible way to slow it down was through hormone treatment.

Then, evolutionary biologists made an interesting theory and decided to test it. The theory was that if the body was stressed continuously even into old age, that the cells of the body would respond to that stress with adaptive growth and repair enabling the cells to continue to function and even grow younger. Along with the cell adaptation, a cascade of enzymes and biological factors would support the growth and repair.

The stress had to be intense and create the micro-tears and strain that heavy, weight-bearing exercise induces.

Of course, any exercise is good for the body at almost any age. But to turn on the repair and adaption mechanisms, it must be intense and weight-bearing. Doing a half an hour on the exercise bike or treadmill is not intense enough. Chair aerobics in the community center will not create the needed strain.

In this case, intense means an elevated heart rate in the 85% to 95% maximum heartbeat range and lasting 40 minutes or more. And, it must be weight-bearing exercise that stresses the bones, ligaments, and tendons as well as the muscles. In testing their theory, they discovered that it does work. And one of the best forms of fitness activity to create that response in the body is Crossfit.

Crossfit takes place in group classes. It is usually in a converted warehouse or commercial facility that has lots of space and height. Crossfit gyms do not have mirrors or machines. They have weights, and barbells, and dumbbells, and kettlebells, and racks used to do weightlifting and floor space to do all kinds of workouts. They have rowers and exercise bikes that are much different than ones usually found in commercial gyms. A class generally consists of some form of weightlifting and then a high intensity interval training -HIIT- workout. A class is usually an hour long. The emphasis is on functional fitness. That is fitness that helps us get through everyday life better.

I know this can sound intimidating and overwhelming… especially if you are out of shape and haven't exercised hard in a long time – or ever. **Please do not think that you must be in shape to get in shape!**

Every workout can be modified for your current level of ability. The coach or coaches can help with alternative movements and weights. It is doable.

Be a beginner. Be open to learning new ways of doing things. Start and go slowly. Push only to the edge a little at a time. As we get older, it takes longer to recover and heal – so do not push over the edge and injure yourself. Follow your coach's directions. Consistency is the key. Show up every day. Doing a little bit more every day is better than trying to do a lot intermittently.

It is really about your intention. It is not about comparing yourself with others. It is about becoming a better version of you today than you were yesterday. And to continue working on that every day. Do you want to be more capable? Do you want to be fitter? Do you want to move better? Do you want to be stronger?

If so, then it is important to buy into the process – the everyday, step by step process of gaining capacity – of gaining mobility – of gaining balance. It means showing up every day.

We will be talking about this much more as we move on. We'll be looking at workouts and how people feel along the path. For now, think about who you want to become and if you are willing to commit to what it takes to get there.

This is the definition – or one of them – that Greg Glassman, the founder and CEO of Crossfit, uses:

> Crossfit is a core strength and conditioning program. We have designed our program to elicit as broad an adaptational response as possible. Crossfit is not a specialized fitness program but a deliberate attempt to optimize physical competence in each of 10 fitness domains. They are cardiovascular/respiratory endurance, stamina, strength, flexibility, power, speed, coordination, agility, balance, and accuracy.
>
> Aside from the breadth or totality of fitness Crossfit seeks, our program is distinctive, if not unique, in its focus on maximizing neuroendocrine response, developing power, cross-training with multiple training modalities, constant training and practice with functional movements, and the development of successful diet strategies.

We will explore this definition of fitness more deeply and expand on the concept in many areas.

Chapter Four

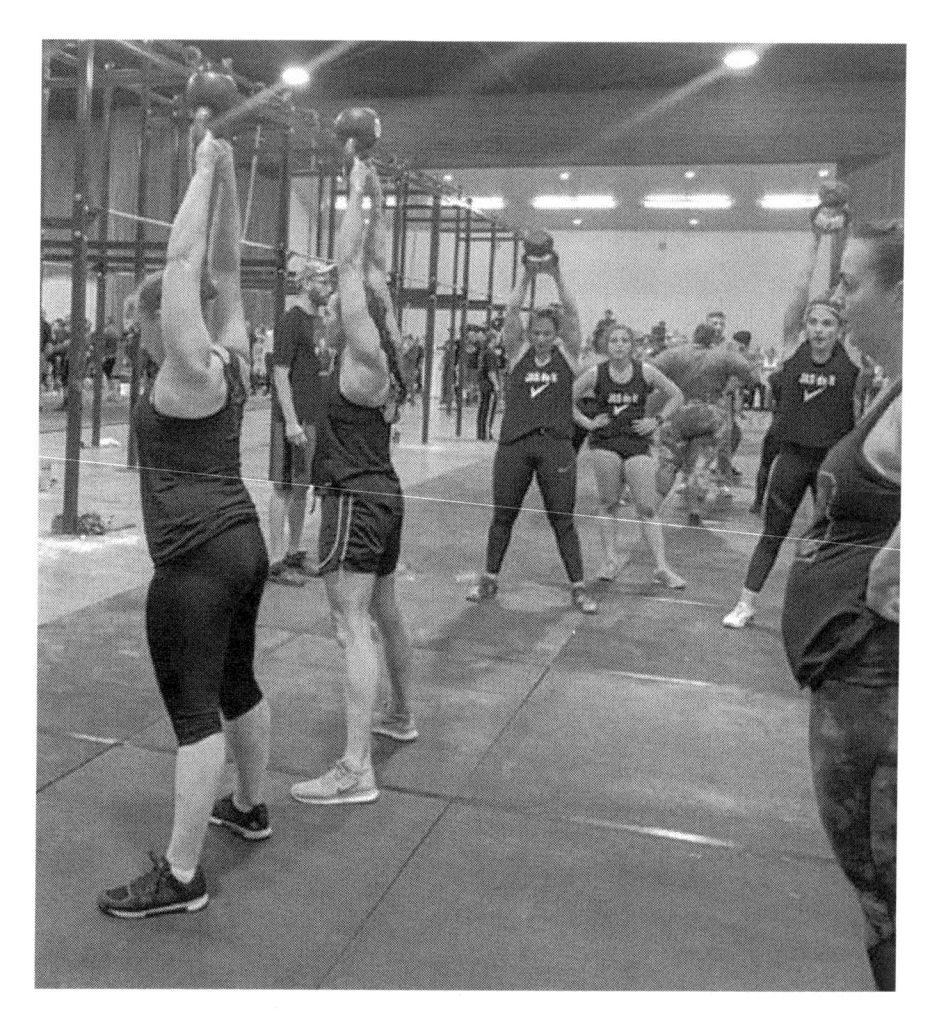

Equally or more important than exercising in becoming an ageless athlete is **nutrition.**

In plain language, your nutrition should consist of garden vegetables (especially greens), meats (non-factory farmed, grass fed) or plant-based protein, nuts and seeds, some fruit, little starch, and no sugar.

Avoid processed food. Avoid high glycemic carbohydrates that raise blood sugar too rapidly. These include rice, bread, candy, potato, sweets, and sodas.

It is just about that simple. It is not easy – but it is simple. We will go into nutrition in more depth later as well.

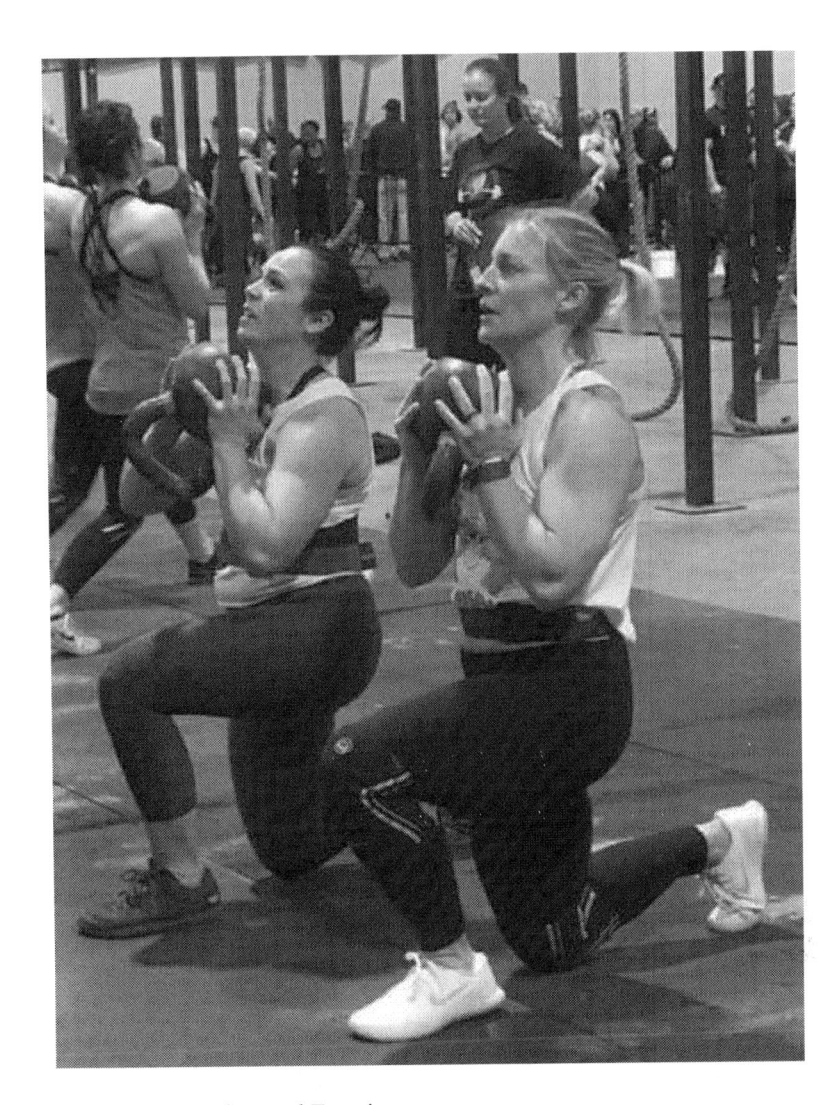

Nutrition, Exercise, and Emotions

We are subject to more stress now than any time in history. Our children have more bits of information thrown at them in a day then their grandparents did in a year. And the amount of fake news, lies, misinformation, propaganda, biased information, opinions, bad news, and exaggerated, dramatized, and misleading information is expanding exponentially every year.

We have no way of knowing what is real, true, and meaningful. Check it on the internet? That is one of the major sources of misinformation.

Children are not taught critical thinking skills and discernment as they once were, so they do not know the questions to ask and the systems of thought needed to determine meaning.

In addition to that, we have learned to manage our stress, and grief, and sadness, and depression, and anxiety, and anger, and uneasiness with food, drink, games, and drugs.

Many of us eat our depression and sadness. Or drink our anger. Or binge our anxiety. Sugar is one of the most abused "drugs" in managing emotions. It becomes programmed into our emotional responses and many of us become addicted to it...or alcohol, or TV, or sex, or risky behavior, or video/computer games.

Unfortunately, older people are more prone to addictive behavior as they age due to loneliness, grief, and illness.

The good news is that exercise and clean eating is a way to positively impact the difficult emotions. Exercise can create endorphins and hormones that help a person have a lighter mood and a more positive outlook. Good nutrition creates a basis for emotional balance and stability.

All the things that we will be discussing in terms of slowing down the aging process also have a positive impact on our emotional life.

The research in this area is well established and clear. Exercise and eat clean. You will feel better. As you get fitter and healthier, you will feel better about yourself. This supports and enhances the feelings generated from exercising and eating well. It is a virtuous circle!

Meditation and Breathing

Another way to relieve stress, mood swings, and other emotional triggers is through breathing and meditation. Emotions are embodied. We carry them in our gut, or muscles, or with clenched teeth, or other ways. Many people carry their anxiety and stress in their necks or upper backs. Some folks clench their fists or teeth when they are angry. We tend to not only carry emotions in our bodies but tend to hold them habitually creating tense and sore places.

Exercise is one way to relieve these kinds of tension. But many times, the emotions are held so deeply and habitually that it takes more than strenuous exercise to reach them. Deep body work like massage or physical therapy may be needed to help relieve that tension. Or, progressive and consistent meditation and breath work.

A simple meditation like breath awareness can work well. Find a room that is darkened, but not black. Sit on the floor on a pillow or cushion. Close your eyes to a slit, but not all the way closed. Start breathing very calmly and slowly, becoming aware of your body, how you are holding it, and where there is tension and stiffness. As you inhale, breath into those areas of tension, and as you exhale, let go of the tension. Don't be in a hurry. Just relax into the breathing.

Your mind will wander. You'll hear sounds outside. You'll have an itch. Your butt will get sore. Just breath and bring your attention back to the tension and letting go. Don't get mad or upset. Just gently bring your attention back to breathing and letting go.

Five or ten minutes at first is enough. Slowly work up to 15 minutes. Letting go. Bringing the attention back to the breath. Every day, if possible, work on this awareness and mediation. Like exercise, it takes time and consistency. It will work and it will help.

Another simple breathing exercise you may like to try is called "Box Breathing." That is not the Sanskrit name for it, but it is handy.

Like before, set up in a darkened room sitting on a pillow or cushion or chair if that is more comfortable. Slowly bring your awareness to your body and your thoughts and emotions. Let them calm down and float without judgement or naming. They are not good or bad...they just are. Floating free and easy.

Bring your awareness to your breath and start to build a box with it:

```
Inhale        1   2   3   4         Hold
4                                    1
3                                    2
2                                    3
1                                    4
Hold          4   3   2   1         Exhale
```

Gently inhale counting to 4. Hold counting to 4. Exhale counting to 4. And hold counting to 4.

Do this three times. And relax. Let go of any tension or stress. Check your body for any stiffness.

Then, do three rounds again. Slowly and gently building a box with your breath. And, relax. Again, let go of any tension or stress remaining.

Then, do it three more times. When you are done, just sit. Let thoughts come and go. Let feelings come and go. Let sensations come and go. No holding. No judging. No grasping. Just easily letting things come and go as they may.

When you are ready, rise and leave the room.

These are just two of many, many meditative and breathing practices. Take a class or watch YouTube. You will not be sorry.

Chapter Five

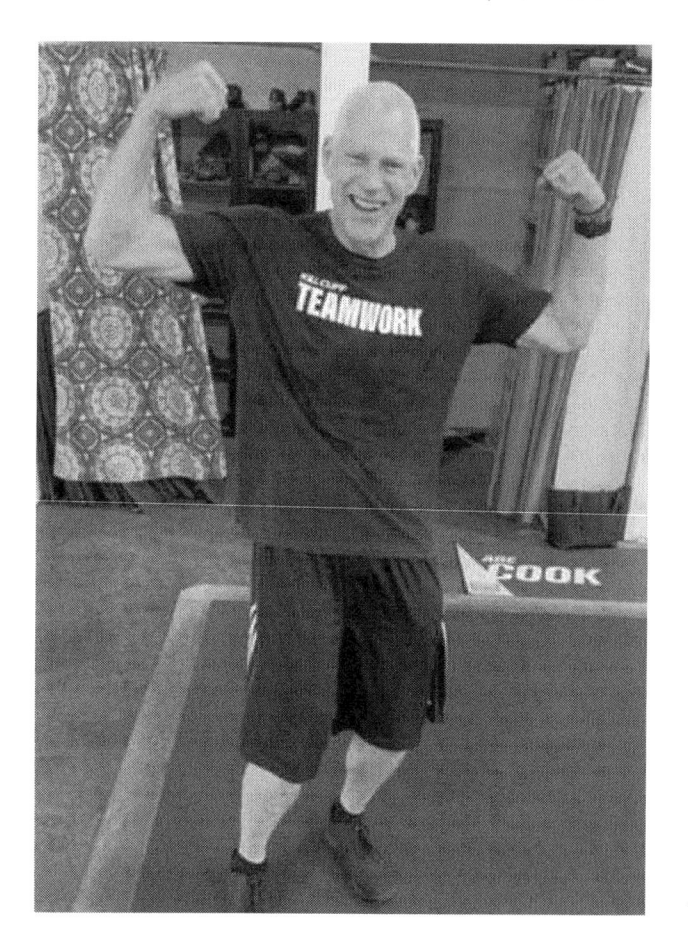

The Aging Athlete's Body

As we age as adults, our bodies go through a constant cycle of compensation and adaptation. We get a sore back playing with our kids. We hold ourselves a certain way to minimize the pain and the chance of doing it again and we adapt the way we move.

We get injured at work. We compensate and adapt. We are ill and we compensate and adapt. We work 40 hours a week at a desk and we compensate and adapt. We drive long hours in our commute or for our work and we compensate and adapt.

Over time, we create a pattern of holding our bodies and adapting the way we move that is restrictive and habitual. We create muscle imbalances and limits to our range of motion. We move generally in one direction – forward – and become uneasy and out of balance when we are forced to move in a different direction.

Our posture changes to accommodate our compensation and restricted movements.

And just like that, we look and feel old.

When we decide to get fit and healthy as older athletes, one of our major battles is regaining mobility and flexibility we lost in our compensation and adaptive processes. We did not build these patterns of posture and imbalances overnight. And we will not correct them overnight.

And, as Brad told me, consistency and focus will allow us to make little advances every day. Over time, big changes will occur.

As an aging athlete, we need to stretch and mobilize every day. I get to the box an hour or 45 minutes early every day, so I have time to warm up and stretch and activate muscles for the workout. I work with a Physical therapist – on and off - who is also a Crossfit athlete, on muscle imbalances. You may not need that much help. A good coach can help tremendously with stretches, warmups, and mobility.

Many people, old and young, just come to the gym, do the warmup on the board for the WOD, and do fine. I need more than that to prepare for the workout.

You can decide once you start working out. Remember, we are looking to do an **intense** workout 4-5 times a week. The intensity is what triggers the repair and adaptive processes that slow down and reverse the aging processes. And good nutrition provides the materials.

So, be prudent. Warm up. Stretch. Mobilize. And listen closely to your body.

Intensity does not mean going 100% all the time for every workout. Please! We would turn into a pile of mush in no time doing that. Intensity means giving the amount of effort to the workout for the purpose it is designed for.

The coach will tell you that this workout is a sprint – all out for 3 minutes, then 3 minutes rest, then all out for 3 minutes, then 3 minutes rest… and so on. Or that the workout is a long one with many movements, so pace yourself and try to have a little reserve to push at the end.

In other words, each workout is different, with different requirements and pacing. The coach will help you determine what that means for you individually. As you get fitter, the definition of intensity will shift. That is part of the fun in Crossfit. You are never done getting fitter and working with more intensity. It is very humbling.

A nice thing about crossfit is that you do not need to figure this out on your own. Every workout and every class has a WOD (workout of the day) prepared for you, with instructions, videos of movements, and coaches to explain the components, pacing, and more.

We come back to these topics many times throughout this book.

Chapter Six

Cross Fit Is Hard

Why so serious?
The Joker

I've been home for almost a week with a blasted summer cold. A couple of folks from the box have contacted me and said I am missed. I've been busy feeling miserable and going into an existential funk.

I've been asking myself if this is the way it will end. When Mr. Death comes up behind me and knocks me down and puts his boot on my neck, is this the way I will go out? Whimpering and complaining like a little baby?

I went to bed last night with the intention of going to my 9 AM class at CFOC this morning. I woke up sweating and coughing and thought one more day at home will probably make all the difference in the world in how I feel. Then I remembered conversations I've had with my friend Astin. She and I talk about "just showing up" a lot and what that means to us. Just show up. Sometimes it is not about motivation. It is just showing up. Sometimes it is hard. Just show up. Sometimes it seems futile. Just show up.

The old Zen saying describes it well: Novice, "Master, before enlightenment what do you do?" Master, "Chop wood. Carry water." Novice, "Master, after enlightenment what do you do?" Master, "Chop wood. Carry water." I'm going to be late.

Astin is there, smiling to see me. She never fails to make me feel better. Sue, Rachel, Gage, Adam, Sarah, all grin hello and wave. Brad notices but doesn't say anything. I don't feel better, but I feel this is where I belong. I warm up, sweat out a 7-minute metcon (metabolic conditioning), then a post-WOD (workout of the day) series of sled pulls, farmers' carries, and shoulder stands. I am dripping by the time I am done. I am glad I came.

I am not a certified coach for crossfit. I am a member of an affiliate. That is it. So, the descriptions of workouts, activities, form, mechanics, movements, and so on are strictly from my perspective and are not the "official" wording or statements from CrossFit.

Crossfit is hard. I never have to worry about getting a good workout. I never have to worry about what muscle group or what movement or what weight I will use. It is all "programmed" for me. I can modify it, with the help of my coach, if I am injured or having mobility issues. As much as I can, I try to do the workouts as described.

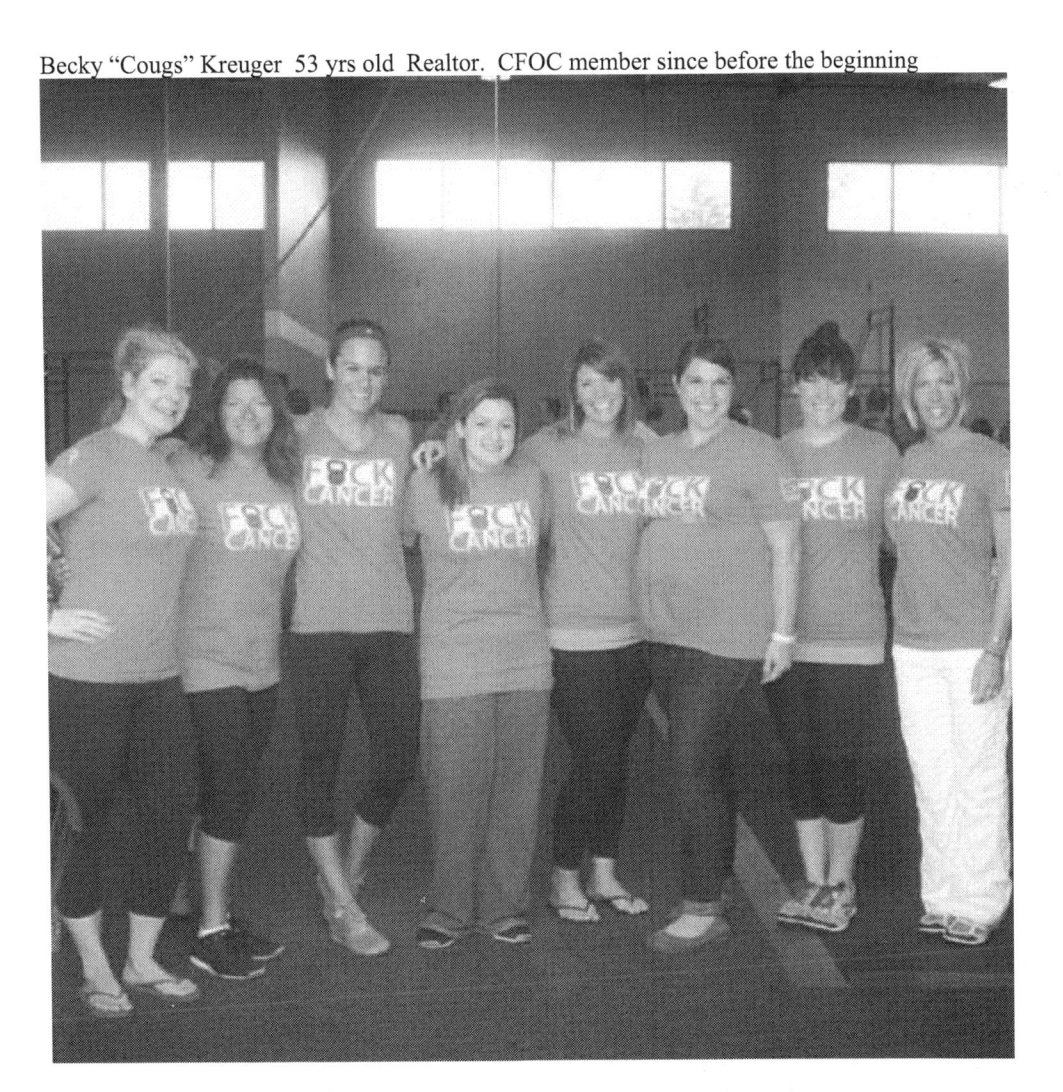

Becky "Cougs" Kreuger 53 yrs old Realtor. CFOC member since before the beginning

If CFOC had membership numbers, Cougs' and her family, Rick and Brianna would be "0". Scott's brother Tony is a close neighbor to the Kreugers. They would often vacation together, and on one Mexican trip, Scott and Jen joined the Kreugers and Tony for a week. Becky and Jen spent the week talking about nutrition and health. Scott and Jen were preparing to move back to Oregon from Texas.

They hit it off and have been close ever since. If there is a model for the relationships that are established in the community at the box, it is the relationship between the Kreugers and the Cereghinos. It is respectful, sassy, loyal, direct, fun, and very, very accepting and supporting.

When Jen and Scott moved, Tony asked the Kreugers to help them get settled and in return Scott and Jen invited them over for a BBQ...a paleo BBQ. After the meal, Jen asked the family into the garage and had everyone do a 5-minute workout. And as they were leaving, Jen said, "11 OK tomorrow?" And they showed up because they were in for helping Scott and Jen any way they could.

Becky had what is kindly called a "rough" childhood. She avoided sports and any activities. When she was older, she joined every gym, and then did not have the nerve to show up. She was anxious when Jen asked them to do the mini workout but she didn't want to say no. The Kreugers went the next day.

Jen kept asking and they kept going – everyday. "Jen, with her stopwatch!" Becky said with a laugh. "I wanted to quit every day." Jen would encourage and push and cajole and Becky would keep coming back. During one workout after a month or so, Becky was jogging, and Jen was talking with her and running backward with her and keeping her occupied, when she realized everyone had stopped and were clapping and cheering. "I looked around and recognized that I had just run my first mile – ever! Jen was so happy for me."

After 2 months in the garage, CFOC officially opened in the warehouse space it still occupies – granted on a much bigger scale. Scott continued to sell oncology imaging equipment on the road to finance the fledgling business while Jen ran the box.

Becky had lung cancer a few years before the Cereghinos moved to Oregon City to start CFOC. She discovered that the cancer returned a year or a year and half after the start of CFOC. There was another member whose house had burned down, and Jen and Scott organized a workout to collect donations to help that member and to collect for an unspecified cancer purpose. Becky jumped right in to help organize the workout and collect donations and to get the community involved. She said, "The whole community showed up. It was awesome!" Two weeks later they honored her with a check to help cover her health care costs. She told me, "I would have worked harder if I had known it was for me." (BTW, CFOC no longer takes direct donations as they did not want to become a 501C3 non-profit. They have other ways of making it work now.)

She and Jen developed a workout plan and nutrition approach to attack the cancer. The tumors stopped growing and then reduced. A few years later, Becky had a heart attack because of the radiation treatment done during her first bout of cancer. She said, "I was so strong I wasn't even sure I was having an attack. I was saved by EMTs and first responders who work out at CFOC!"

Becky says that she and her family are perfect examples of what crossfit can do for people. "I am a cancer survivor. I can lift my baggage into the overhead bin on an airplane, then help others. I do slow, proper form with beautiful movements. It translates into everyday life. My daughter has lost 75 pounds. I am so lucky. This is so fun! This is family."

Now is a good time to get back to **Nutrition.**

Cancer, diabetes, dementia and heart disease are a few of the chronic diseases that strike more often as we age. Along with the body losing strength and bones getting weaker, aging causes the immune system and other disease-fighting mechanisms to diminish. The story is like what we were told about muscle strength and bones – it is inevitable and progressive.

And, like the story about muscles, it is not the whole story and there are things that can be done to slow the process and even reverse it in some areas.

Nutrition is a topic that has more contradictions, misinformation, false claims, and half-truths than just about any other health topic. We are inundated with articles and advertising for organic this, and natural that, and enriched, and gluten-free, and fortified, and grass-fed, and more. And it seems to change every week.

Let's set the record straight based on nutritional science as it stands today. Just as with exercise, this is not about a "diet." It is about a lifestyle!

In order to give your body the kind of fuel it needs to repair and grow the cells that are stressed each day by strenuous exercise you must create an eating plan based on whole foods. No processed food of any kind.

Let's talk about what you can't eat first if you want to slow down or reverse aging.

NO!
Soda/pop
Sugar
Alcohol
Red meat
Processed meat
Starches – potatoes, rice, pasta
Grains – doesn't matter if whole grains or not
Packaged cereal, pre-packaged meals, ketchup, peanut butter, and more.
Dairy

If you are like me, you are amazed by some of the things on this list. There are more items to consider, but we will discuss what these items have in common first.

Meats that come from the factory farms of the US are loaded with things that cause rapid aging and bad health. If you consider matter to be information – atoms, molecules, etc., as quantum scientist do- then the information contained in red meat from these farms is contaminated with mis-spelled words, bad punctuation, gibberish, and more. It causes a lot of damage to occur over time in the body's cells. Foremost among those damages is causing the body to get fat. Next is inflammation. And finally, there is cell destruction. Factory farm meat is grain fed, has antibiotics and steroids in it, and is slaughtered and packaged under horrible conditions. Just consider the number of E. Coli outbreaks in the past few years as an indication of those conditions.

Red meat – beef and pork – and white meat -chicken and turkey – are equally suspect. If you must eat meat, the order of worst to not so bad goes from factory farm red meat, grass fed red meat, factory farm white meat, free range white meat, then fish, to oil-rich fish. The best source of protein is plant-based sources.

The typical American's diet consists of red meat, potatoes, and grain products sweetened with a lot of sugar. It is impossible to stay healthy and fit with this diet. Period.

Sugar is as bad as any street drug on the market. It is more addictive than crack-cocaine. It is one of the most inflammation-causing substances known. It doesn't matter whether it is sucrose, dextrose, or fructose. They all cause enormous damage. The Big Food industry of the West has done a wonderful job of turning us all into sugar junkies. And our health and aging processes pay the price.

As I said at the beginning of this book, don't take my word for it. Do your own research and due diligence. We've been conned for a long, long time. And the misinformation out to the public is worse than the tobacco industry ever tried to feed us. The food pyramid that is used to create a "healthy" diet is pure propaganda. Who benefits? The food industry, big pharma, health care companies, the diet industry and more. We eat a diet that results in obesity, diabetes, heart disease, cancer, dementia and more. Then we are told all we must do is diet and exercise and it will go away. Yes, that is partially true, but not at all like what we've been hearing for years and years.

They (meaning the food industry et al) want to make it our fault that we have fat kids and can't stay on a diet for long. When we do manage to lose weight, it is only a short time before we gain it back and more. And we feel guilty and inadequate because we can't do it. That is not the case.

The food we are eating -meat based protein, grains, sugars, starches – is almost perfectly designed like a biological weapon to keep us over-weight, sluggish, lethargic, and lacking energy. And it is full of addictive substances.

No wonder we can't get healthy and stay fit. In addition, all those foods help accelerate aging and create openings for the chronic diseases we talked about earlier.

We will get into more detail about creating a healthy lifestyle that includes good nutrition and the right kind of exercise as we move along. This is just the beginning.

Let's talk more about exercise and Crossfit now.

Crossfit is hard. And you may want to quit every day. And you will keep coming back because you are surrounded by people who have made the same choices you have – to get a little more fit each day. It is those people in your class who support you, hold you accountable and suffer with you through every workout.

You do not need to be fit to start crossfit. That would be like taking guitar lessons, so you could take guitar lessons. You start where you are. And coaches and the programming and the members all help you figure it out. All you do is show up. And sweat!

Doing the workout as described can take many different forms. The coach or coaches go over the workout at the beginning of each class. They talk about the movements, demonstrate good form, talk about the intensity level the workout is designed for and what kind of pacing makes sense. They take questions and then start the warmup.

I come early almost every day as I need extra time to warmup. I have some mobility and flexibility drills to do as well as hip activation and shoulder activation drills. I am usually (always) sore from the previous day's workout.

Sore is not bad. Hurt is bad. Sore is the body letting you know that you pushed some muscles, tendons and joints into growing and changing. Sore is the signal that good stuff is happening. I welcome sore. And, after a good warmup I don't feel sore.

Then we start the workout. Today it is a partner AMRAP (As Many Reps As Possible). Run 400m together then 10 rounds of Chief alternating partners after each round. Chief is 3 power cleans, 6 hand release pushups and 9 air squats. After 10 rounds we run again. Tina and I complete 24 rounds. It was plenty intense, and I am dripping sweat when we stop.

This type of workout stresses being able to move weight and bodyweight over time and when fatigued. It builds stamina and endurance. It is High Intensity Interval Training, as each partner gets a short rest while the other completes a round. It kicks my butt and I love it.

A year ago, when I started, I would have needed to stop many times during the workout to catch my breath. Today I was able to complete each round unbroken (no stopping) for the entire workout. There is great satisfaction in that. After the workout, many folks stay around for a while to talk, while the 10 0'clock class filters in and starts warming up.

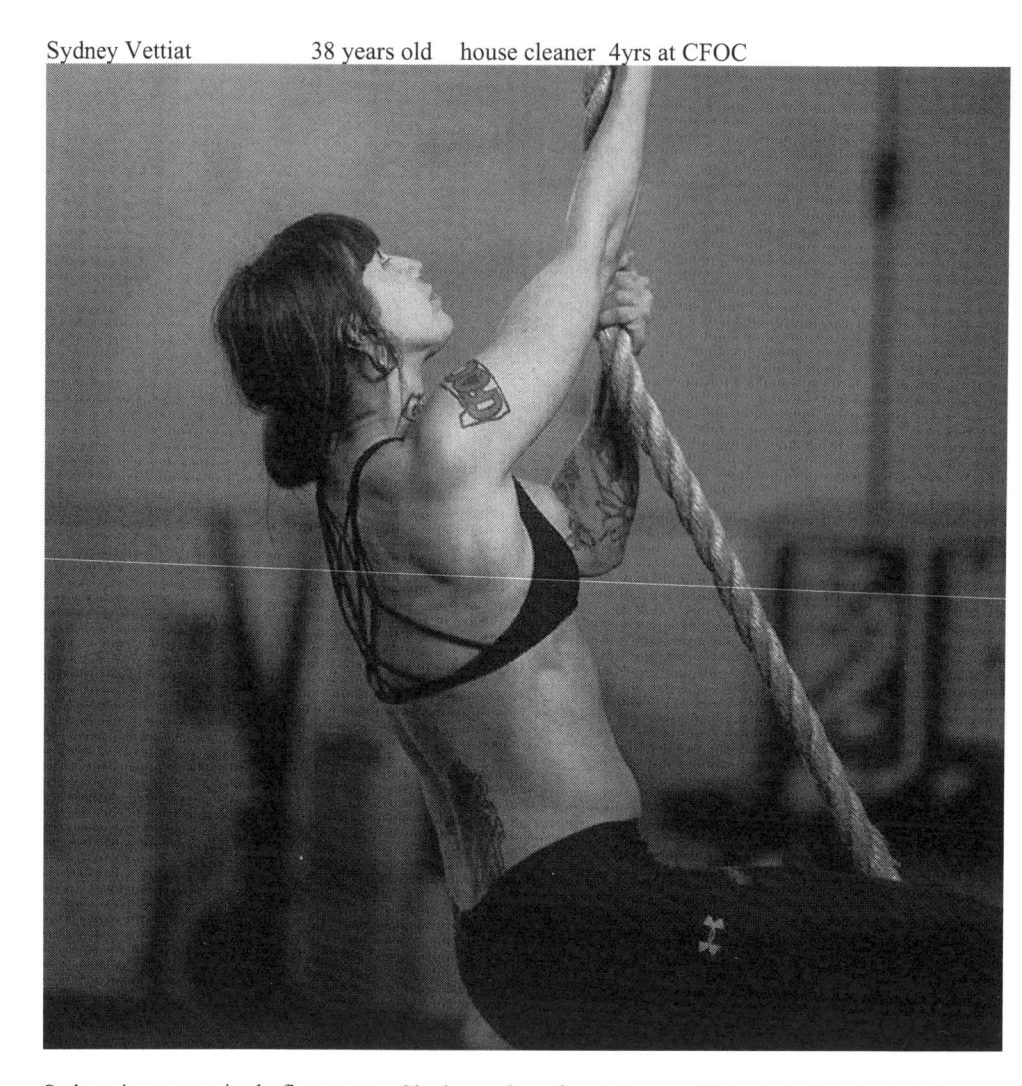

Sydney Vettiat	38 years old	house cleaner 4yrs at CFOC

Sydney is an amazingly fit woman. She has quite a few tattoos and blue hair (It is back to her natural shade now). She has that "crossfit" air of confidence and strength that women seem to gain very quickly here. She tells me that her early years included making a lot of poor decisions as well as getting into some pretty crazy relationships. Her marriage was a mess and her life seemed out of control. She knew something had to change. She came to CFOC to see if she might be interested. She was totally intimidated by the ripped women she saw.

Then she met Jen. She says that is when her life started to change. She started gaining self-confidence. She started seeing healthy relationships. She decided she needed to get a divorce and move on with a more positive set of goals and people in her life.

She said, "It can be the darkest of darkest days – and at the end of the day I can go to cross fit! CFOC saved my life!"

The community accepted and welcomed her. No judgements. She made friends with Emily, who took her under her wing and shared everything she could to help. It made her feel like she was not a duck but could become a swan. Her negative self-image changed. And her life changed.

"I have a life of positivity and brightness. I have discipline and respect. No judgment at all. It is family."

"Here, people make it OK to grow, to change, to challenge yourself, to push your limits. I feel sorry for people who don't come here. It is so safe. It is so warm. It is home."

She says there are so many benefits above and beyond the physical that it is hard to describe.

"Everyone here has a drive to be healthy. We connect through that."

Yes, crossfit is hard. And it yields great benefits.

Crossfit is not for everyone. I know that may come as a shock, but crossfit is not like many other organizations in the fitness industry where they want you to sign up as a member but hope that you will not show up to use the equipment. Crossfit knows that you will not benefit as much by coming once or twice a week. Crossfit is built around a 5-day model – 5 days working out with 2 rest days interspersed. Cross fit knows that doing endless cardio while listening to your tunes is not the recipe for success. Crossfit knows that many folks do not want to work as hard as it takes to be fit. And that is OK.

Crossfit is built on varied, functional movements. Which means that it is transferable to everyday life…picking up the baby or grandchild from the floor, placing baggage or items overhead, moving heavy objects over time (loading a moving van), shoveling snow, and so on.

There are a lot of law enforcement officers, firefighters, first responders, and military personnel who are members of CFOC. They often talk about how cross fit is the best type of fitness training for their jobs because of the movements, varied intensity and length, strength training, and more.

It can be intimidating walking onto a box for the first time. There are no mirrors. There are no weight machines. There is a lot of open space with rubber matting on the floor, some rowing machines, airdynne bikes (devil bikes!), ropes hanging from the ceiling, and racks and benches used for pullups, muscle-ups, and weightlifting movements. Then, there are a bunch of barbells against the wall, followed by row after row of stacked weight plates. And, against another wall is a large set of racks for dumbbells and kettlebells, some that are insanely heavy.

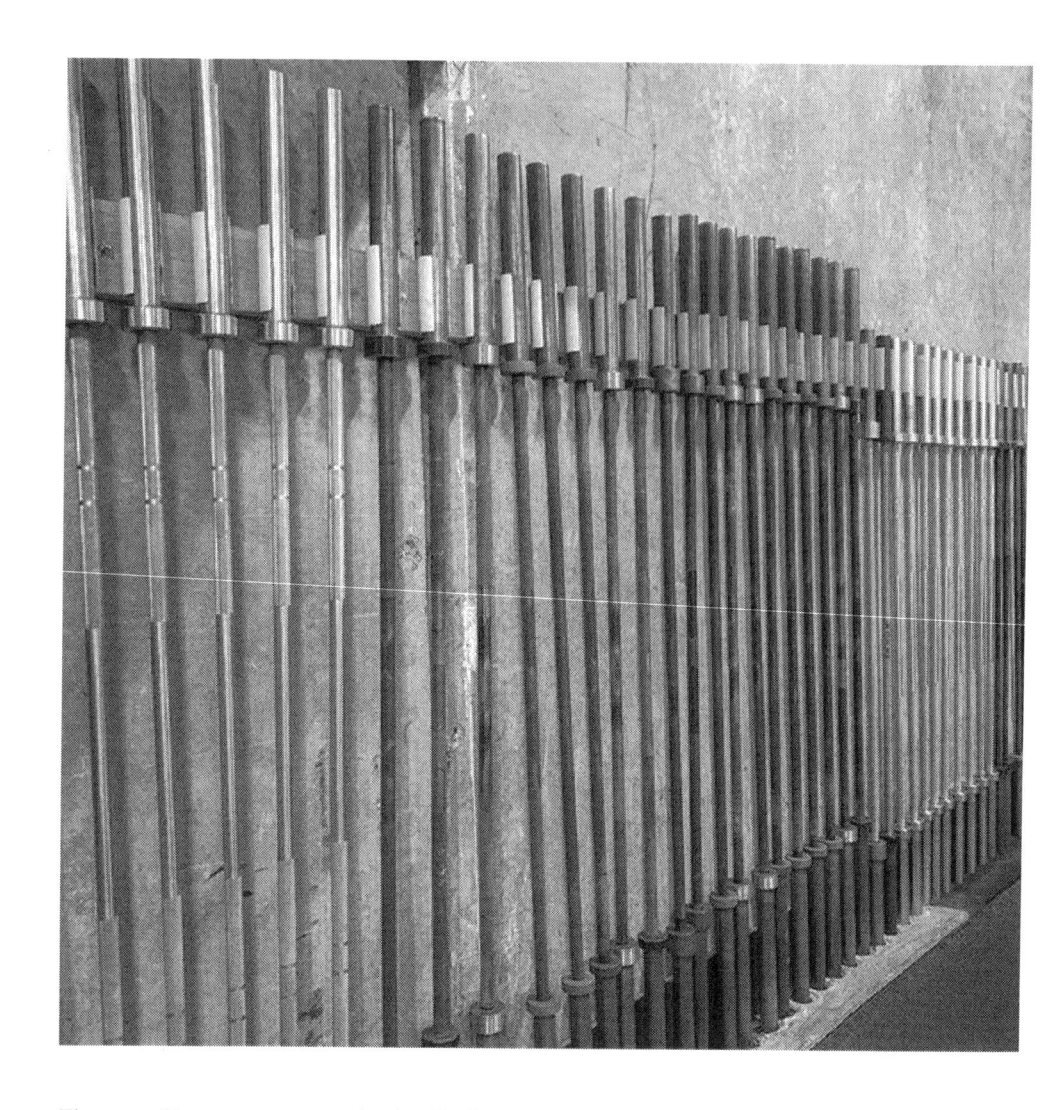

They say, "Leave your ego at the door" when starting crossfit. That is awfully hard to do when you've spent years establishing yourself as an expert, a master, an authority, a competent person in some difficult field and now some "gym instructor" wants you to leave your ego outside? Right....

As the story with Brad illustrated, even those who are experts in fitness may have something to learn from crossfit. I certainly did.

My self-awareness was not particularly accurate when it came to my fitness level and abilities. Scott met me the first day and said that he would be working out with me and that we would follow the workout – or not – depending how well I was able to do the movements. We listened as Brad explained the workout. I was introduced as the "new guy" which was about as pleasant as being introduced in Jr. High as the new student. Then we warmed up.

The workout included barbell work. Scott took one look at me, with my rounded shoulders, caved in chest, head thrust forward posture, and said, "You've been working at a desk most of your life, haven't you?" I had to admit that was true. He said that I would have mobility and flexibility issues because of that so we would start slowly with movements that did not require big changes in my posture.

Instead of a barbell, he got two dumbbells and showed me how to do the movements. I felt stiff as a board and it was hard to get into the right positions. Scott said not to worry. With work, it would come. What an understatement!

After 5 or so months, one of my first coaches – Josh – came to me before he left to go work at a friend's gym. He said, "Todd, I wish I had a picture of you when you walked through the door for the first time. You were a bent over old man. Now, look at you!" And he was right. I felt completely different than I had. I moved differently. I was stronger. I had more stamina. My posture was totally improved. And I have continued to make amazing changes. Just show up!

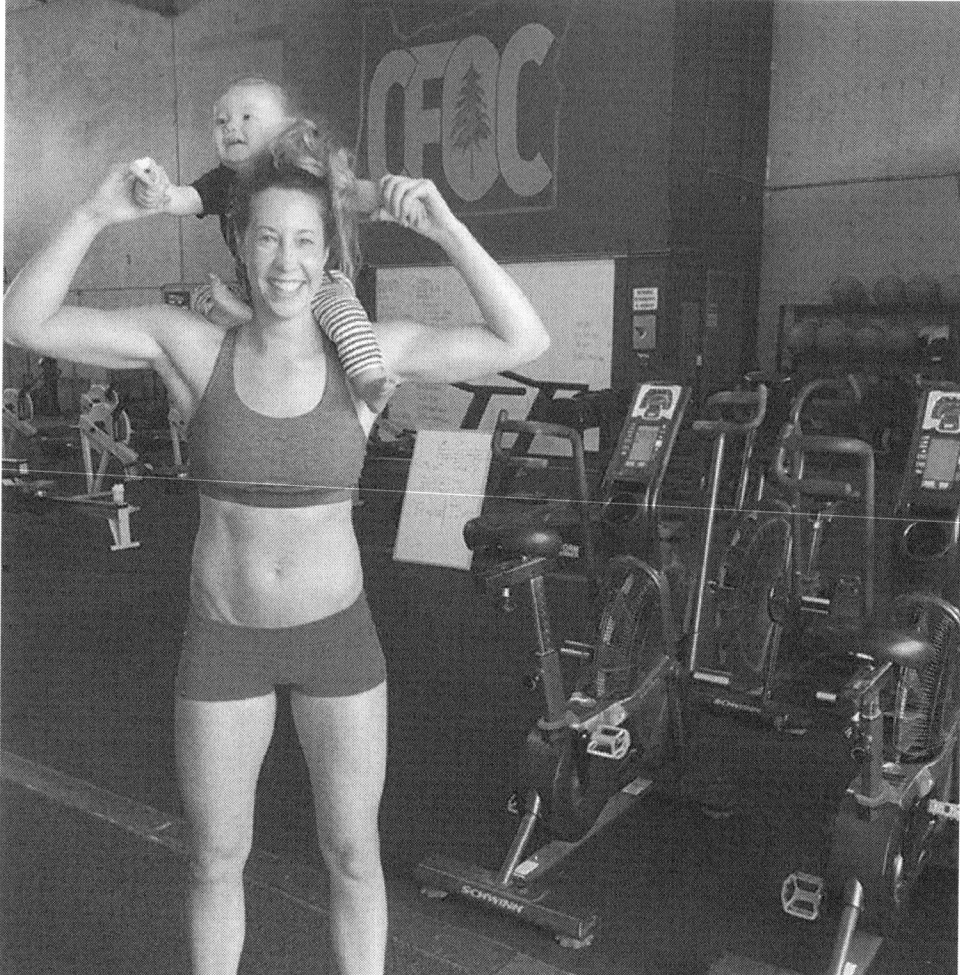

Emily Roberts   31 yrs old   cross fit coach and personal trainer

    Emily is a tall stunning athlete. She moves with the grace of a trained dancer and is stronger than most of the men in the box. She grew up in a competitive, sports-oriented household with 6 siblings. Her dream was to be a pro basketball player.

    Due to ankle injuries she was unable to pursue her basketball dreams. She went to college to become a fitness instructor. Emily started working at a Nautilus training center and enjoyed teaching classes and doing personal training. One day at the grocery store, she ran into Dani, who used to work at Nautilus. Dani had started working out and training at CFOC and told Emily she needed to check it out. She went the following Monday and it has been 4 years as a member and coach since then.

    She was intimidated at first. She didn't know the "language" of crossfit, and the intensity was much different than what she was used to. She said that compared to the other women she felt out of shape. Dani helped a lot and then Jen started coaching her as she wanted to do a competition later that summer.

Here is how Emily described her experience with Jen:
> It is the most I ever learned. She taught me to fuel myself better. She taught me when to moderate when I had setbacks. She taught me how to train my ankles. It was the hardest work I have ever done and the most rewarding. Jen saved my life.
>
> My marriage was falling apart. I was not confident. Jen started working with me and taught me what it means to be an athlete. She taught me what it means to be a woman and what I deserve and that I should not settle for less. She sets such a great example of what it can be like. She is an example of what I can be!
>
> This is such a safe place. There is no judgement. It is like a family.

I talked later with Jen and Emily about this conversation. I also talked with every female member of CFOC who agreed to be interviewed about elements of this conversation. The results of those conversations will be discussed in the section called "The Women of CFOC."

I used Emily and Brad as examples of how much a person can learn when they let go of what they already know. I tell anybody who will listen that one of the best aspects of crossfit for me is that I feel like a kid. I am learning so much. I am having so much fun. I am challenged every day to grow is some new way. I am surrounded by people who are doing the same thing and sharing and laughing and crying together as we do it. How does it get better than this?

After today's workout I was talking with the "other" Todd A. Weber about how things are going with the writing and what I was working on. It is amazing how invested the members are in this book. They want it to relate the significance and importance the box and the community plays in their lives. They want me to get it "right." Todd asked how going over the interviews and writing made me feel. I said it was motivating and inspiring. And, I said, it is a reminder of how grateful I am that I found this place.

Todd replied, "Maybe that is the special sauce."

Chapter Seven

Community

There is a lot of research that indicates that being connected to a community is greatly beneficial to our health. It is even more important as we age. Good relationships and belonging to something meaningful to us helps regulate our emotional state. Like exercise it also helps reduce depression.

I set out to explore what made the Crossfit community so unique. As I got deeper into the process it became apparent that it is like peeling an onion. Each new layer reveals another.

I looked for the "dark side" of the community as well. Trained as I am, I know that it is the shadow side of communities that hold the juicy, dramatic, secretive aspects that give many people satisfaction in belonging. Crossfit is not without some shadowy corners, but they are amazingly harder to discern and have little if any impact on how people relate…or less so than in most communities.

Crossfit has been called a cult by some in the media and parts of the fitness field. People who join boxes can tend to get so excited that all they can talk about is crossfit. If crossfit has a component that is different, special, unique, or magical it is the community that forms in the boxes. If it is a cult (and I don't think it is) it is a healthy one.

Not all boxes form good, healthy communities. Many members of CFOC came from other boxes where the dynamics are much different. Many members of CFOC travel often and visit other boxes when they do. They report that in general most boxes are friendly and welcoming. They also report that there is a wide disparity in cleanliness, equipment maintenance, quality of coaching, and appearance of the boxes.

Since the operating model for crossfit affiliates seems to be a relatively loose set of guidelines, it is not surprising there would be quite a variation in how boxes function. Again, I am not part of crossfit in any way other than as a member of an affiliate. I do not know what affiliates are required to do to become an affiliate and to remain one. I do not know what governing or regulating processes if any that crossfit has to track affiliates. My sense is that affiliate owners are left with a lot of latitude with how they do business and what standards they choose to maintain. It is up to the market to determine who is doing it right. And up to the consumer to look around for a better fit, if the first one does not work.

For the older athlete, community is hugely important in many ways. Moving towards fitness and health with the crossfit workouts provides opportunities for bonding with other members. In our effort and fatigue and struggles and pain and the successes and gains, we create friendships and connections that are extraordinarily strong.

We learn about peoples' families and jobs, where their kids go to school, about their struggles with weight or illness. We go out for coffee together or for a meal after workouts. We BBQ together and create social events together.

We grow close.

Part of the dynamic is suffering through the workouts together. We share the pain and effort. It creates an openness and sharing that is powerful. We share a common belief about the importance of health and fitness that provides a firm foundation.

We get to know people at a deeper level, and it allows us to be more accepting and supporting. When things like differing political opinions come up, we have a foundation of trust and acceptance and we don't have to be triggered. We generally listen with respect, or make jokes, or indicate indirectly or subtly that there is a difference in opinion. Usually that is the end of it.

And often there is a deeper dynamic occurring. Part of crossfit is an exploration of self. We explore the limits of our stamina, and strength, and mental discipline. We are pushing to grow, so we become aware of our limits in many ways – not all of which are physical.

We learn to accept some limits as permanent (for now) and others as subject to change with work and discipline and consistency. And we learn how that may apply to other aspects of our lives.

Aging athletes may have an advantage in that we may already be exploring aspects of our mortality as get closer to death. Physical limits are part of that. Exploring other aspects like our shadow side in another.

In aging, we have the chance to accept the paradox of being human more clearly. We know we are not just one thing or just one kind of person. We tell the truth and we lie. We are trustworthy and we betray. We are loyal and we are fickle. We are brave and we are cowards.

We may not have accepted or become fully aware of those paradoxes. As we age and ask the questions about whether we've lived an authentic life, we must get honest with ourselves. Did I live to please others and their idea of what a good life means? Did I take control of my own destiny? Or, did I, like most people do some of both as well as other dynamics?

In examining these questions, we are faced with some choices. How am I going to live out the time left to me? What are the choices I will make today that will move me in the direction I want to grow? Who am I becoming and how do I keep moving in that direction?

For me, crossfit provides a model for finding some answers.

When I faced the realization that I was "that guy" in the airport that others would not want to sit next to, I could have decided, "F%ck them. I am going home to Oreos, ice cream, and Tacos." Or, many other choices. Instead, I chose to move toward health and quality of life. Obviously, my biases and beliefs are reflected in that choice – but I had not been living up to them.

Now that I am more aligned with my health and fitness goals, where else am I "pretending" or unaware of being out of alignment? Where else have I been coasting passively toward death instead of trying to keep growing, learning, and contributing?

I know the story about aging I had was untrue. What other stories am I living that I can change?

There is a lot to examine. And to make choices for action from here on out.

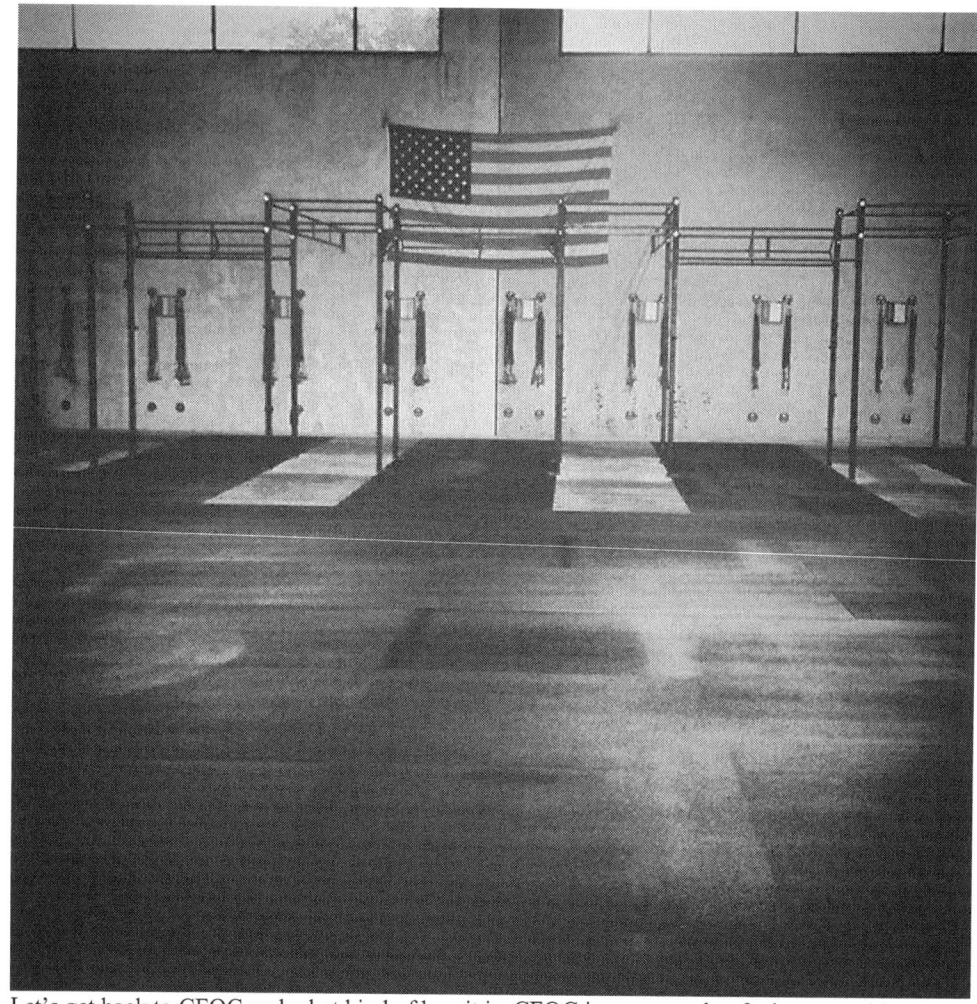

Let's get back to CFOC and what kind of box it is. CFOC is an example of what a good box should be, I think. It is clean… exceptionally clean. The equipment is well cared-for and maintained. The restrooms are kept clean. The play area for the children is clean. Folks are encouraged to wipe down equipment they use and return it to where it belongs. Folks who finish a workout before others often stick around to help with returning weights and equipment. There is a sense of pride and ownership members have in the appearance and cleanliness of the box.

In this time of COVID-19, the box is kept extremely clean and sanitized. Workout spaces are marked out in tape. Any equipment, weights, bars, or dumbbells are cleaned and sanitized before being put back. The whole gym is cleaned between classes.

As is the case with all businesses, the tone is set by the owners. Jen and Scott are passionate about CFOC and crossfit. It shows in everything they do. Every detail is thought out. There is an intentionality to every aspect of CFOC that I did not genuinely appreciate until I had a chance to interview the owners for this book.

CFOC attracts a membership that is somewhat homogenous. It is middle- to upper middle-class and probably slightly older than most commercial gyms. The people here are "doers." They own small businesses. They are law enforcement and fire fighters. They are educators. They are nurses and professionals. They got to where they are today through hard work. Not one of the people I've met at CFOC has a whiff of entitlement. It is apparent that they are willing to put in hard work to get where they want to go.

They are non-judgmental and accepting. Not blindly so, but with the understanding that we'll reach out to help if you are willing to help yourself as well. There is no creed or gospel or manifesto that one must agree to in order to become a member of crossfit. There are Republicans, Democrats, Presbyterians, Catholics, and Rama Krishnas in the community. However, there are core values that are the foundation of the community that are unspoken, but non-negotiable.

One of the things I found most enjoyable about becoming a part of this community is how the members reach out to accept and embrace you almost immediately. They are helpful. They want you to feel welcome. They know it can be intimidating. And they want you to stick around long enough to get a good sense of crossfit before you decide if it is a good fit.

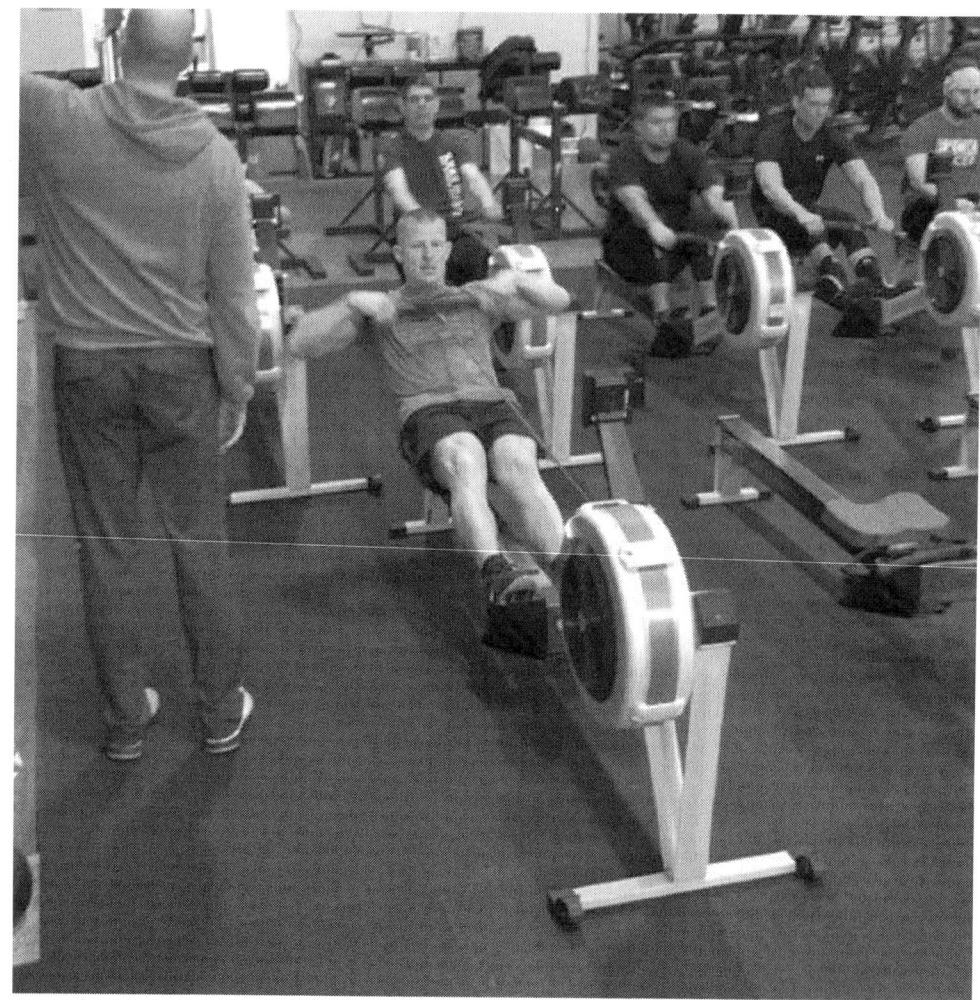

I may describe these foundations differently than what is intended, as I am trying to make written what are unwritten rules.

Number one is simple and direct. You work for what you get. There is no magic pill. If you want to get fit, do the work. If you want to join this community start sweating. The members are welcoming, accepting, and non-judgmental. And they will watch. Are you willing to get your hands dirty? Do you complain too much about a workout? Are you negative? Do you support others when they need it? Are you a loner, or are you a part of the team? Do you gossip?

Number two is also simple. Everybody helps. We pick up after ourselves. We help watch the kids. We help the new people. We help clean up. We are self-sufficient.

Number three is a little more complex. We give back when we can. As a group, we understand how fortunate we are. We worked for it AND we had good fortune along the way. Not that this group has not had tragedy, grief, loss, and misfortune. It has. It is through those losses and tragedies that we've come to appreciate what we have even more. And it is through those losses that we've gained a better understanding of what it means to give and support when we can.

I'll be discussing the many ways that CFOC gives back to the community and supports its members later. It is part of the fabric of this community and Crossfit as a whole.

I asked Jen and Scott if they ever had to kick out a member. They said yes – twice.

One was a person who created safety issues for himself and others. He would not listen when advised to use less weight and work on form. He insisted on pushing beyond what he was capable of and in the process created potential for injury to himself and others. The coaches and Jen and Scott asked him and then told him on multiple occasions to ease back a bit. He refused. They asked him to leave.

The other was a person so negative she was creating a problem. Nothing was ever right. The workout was wrong. The coaches weren't helping. The equipment didn't work. Her partner distracted her. The music was too loud. It went on and on. Again, Jen and Scott and the coaches tried to inform her of the issue and hoped she would change. She did not.

Jen and Scott told me that most people self-select to become members of the box. Usually, within three or four workouts, a person can tell if it is a fit. And they can tell if they will be able to do and enjoy the workouts. It tends to draw people who are willing to work and push themselves out of their comfort zones. As I mentioned before, the work gets done on the edges of comfort zones. The edge for Crossfit is about doing more than you thought you could, pushing harder than you thought possible, finishing that last minute or two of a workout when all you want to do is quit. That is where we become fitter, build more capacity, and grow.

Crossfit is more than physical. It requires mental discipline and emotional stamina. As you get fitter and stronger, those elements become even more important.

The members are the folks who challenged authority in school and then became authority figures. They are used to getting things done. They push themselves to be better every day and they expect that you are there for the same reasons. That is not to say that everything is serious and clenched jaw. Far from it. People in this community have a lot of fun together. They are masters at teasing each other and smack-talking just the right amount to get a better performance out of each other. They are competitive, but not destructive or hurtful about it. They want to see each other do their best – in everything.

The more competitive folks tend to bunch together during workouts and those who are more into pushing their limits individually bunch together. There is a togetherness that binds us all. And there is support and encouragement for all.

Gage and Rachel Halland 39, 36

Gage and Rachel are some of my favorite people. They are young parents of two boys who bring a lively openness to all that they do. Gage is a luthier -acoustic guitar maker. His guitars are works of art. Rachel is a HR/operations specialist.

Gage's dad was an athlete and coach and taught Gage to be highly active when he was young. They didn't have TV in the home so he would be outside with his friends being active all day.

Rachel grew up doing water sports and boating. Her parents were very conservative in teaching Rachel about being an athlete (she shouldn't be one was the message) so she had some internal battles to overcome when deciding to get fit.

They tried CFOC about 5 years ago for one class and didn't like it. They said it was really intimidating and humbling. Soon after, they left for Quebec where Gage had a two-year internship with a master luthier.

Gage's dad had a heart attack when he was healthy and Gage thought that if that could happen, what were his odds? He and Rachel got involved in P90 workouts at home and tried other systems to get strong and fit.

They moved back to Portland and met some parents of kids at their sons' school who were at CFOC and decided to try it again. They paid for 3 months in advance so they would not back out of it.

The first two weeks were humbling and awfully hard. But they decided they liked the challenge and made it into a "date night" approach. They liked doing the partner WODS together and they both were blown away by Sarah! They said that she is so strong and fit that it is amazing and they both wanted to be like her.

Rachel was fighting through a challenge about how strong women "should" be and decided that she was going to break through that barrier. They both made tremendous gains quickly. Rachel started competing and Gage started hanging out with some of the stronger members. Rachel said that she began to understand how strong she could be and liked it.

Both Gage and Rachel have a great sense of humor and are a great deal of fun to hang out with. Unfortunately, they decided to move to Montana where Gage could build his shop more affordably, so we don't have them around anymore.

I miss them a lot.

Chris and Rose Lambert   53 & 50   business owners

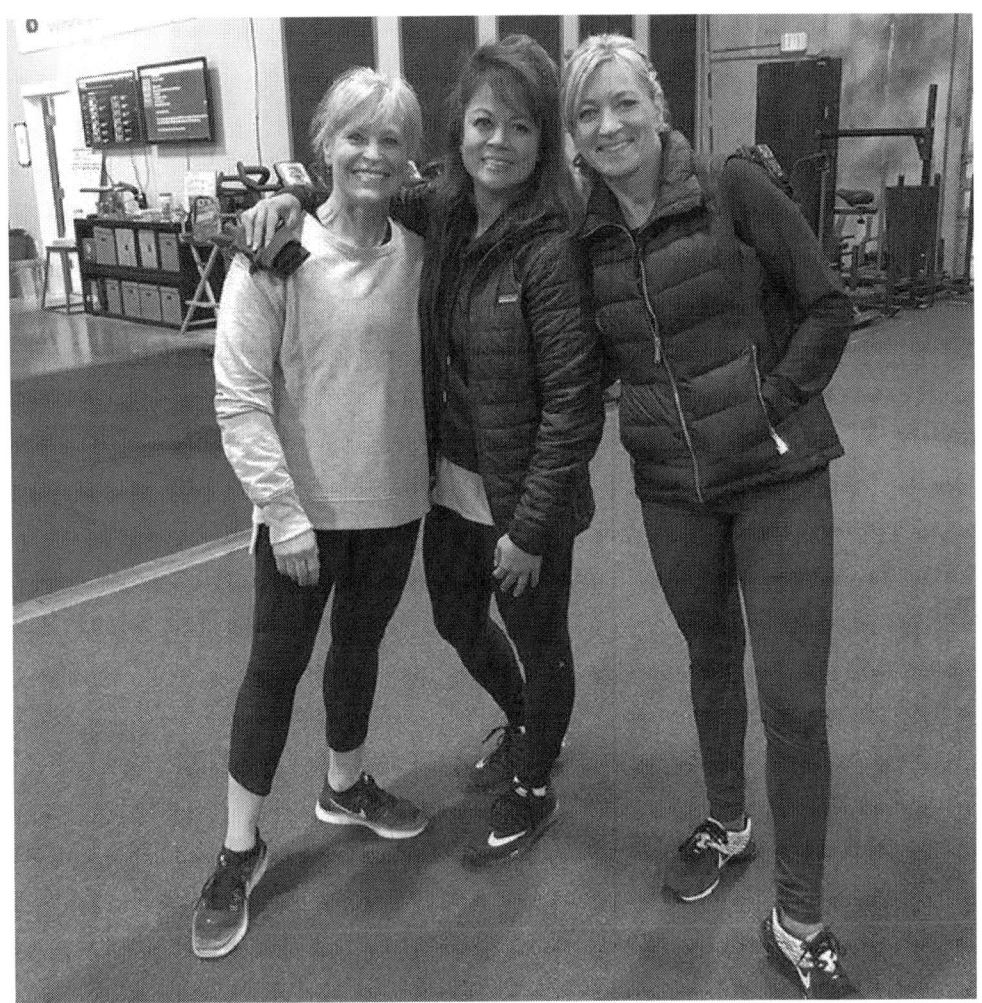

Chris and Rose are a very engaging and enjoyable couple. They tend to finish each other's sentences and laugh a lot. They ran into Dani about 5 years previously and she told them about CFOC. They said it took a while, but they finally joined. They were introduced to Jen and Scott and did the first workout. As Chris described it, it was ridiculously hard. The next day was miserable – beyond normal.

Both agreed that they had been deluding themselves about how fit they were and that they knew it was time to get to work. They never felt judged or criticized. No one is here to show somebody up. Leave your stuff at the door and get to work.

They said they have never met someone as committed as Jen. People are first and the business is second for her. Oh, and Scott too ?

Everybody is real, wide open, honest and humble. It took a while to make friends, they said, but now their whole social life is centered on people at the box. Rose stated that she loves what it does for her everyday life! Every day I say a secret thank you to crossfit.

Chris and Rose echo what almost everyone I interviewed said about the people at CFOC. Folks are authentic, open, sharing, non-judgmental, caring and respectful. There are many, many differences, and people accept them all.

The classes at CFOC start at 5 AM during the week and the last one is at 6:30 PM or later. On Saturday, the official class is at 9, but there are early groups and a lifting class at 10 most Saturdays. People tend to hang out more on Saturdays catching up with folks from different classes and letting the kids have some fun together.

There is open gym during the middle of the day usually and on Sundays. There are some differences between the classes. Some of it is due to who coaches each class normally and some of it is due to the makeup of the members who are regulars to that class.

You tend to get to know the people in your class the best. There are a bunch of folks who go to different classes, particularly during the summer, but I would say for the most part, people seem to be creatures of habit.

Saturday workouts and the special workouts are where people get together more as a whole community. There is a special energy in the box when 100 or more people are doing the same workout together. There is a buzz and connection that seems magical.

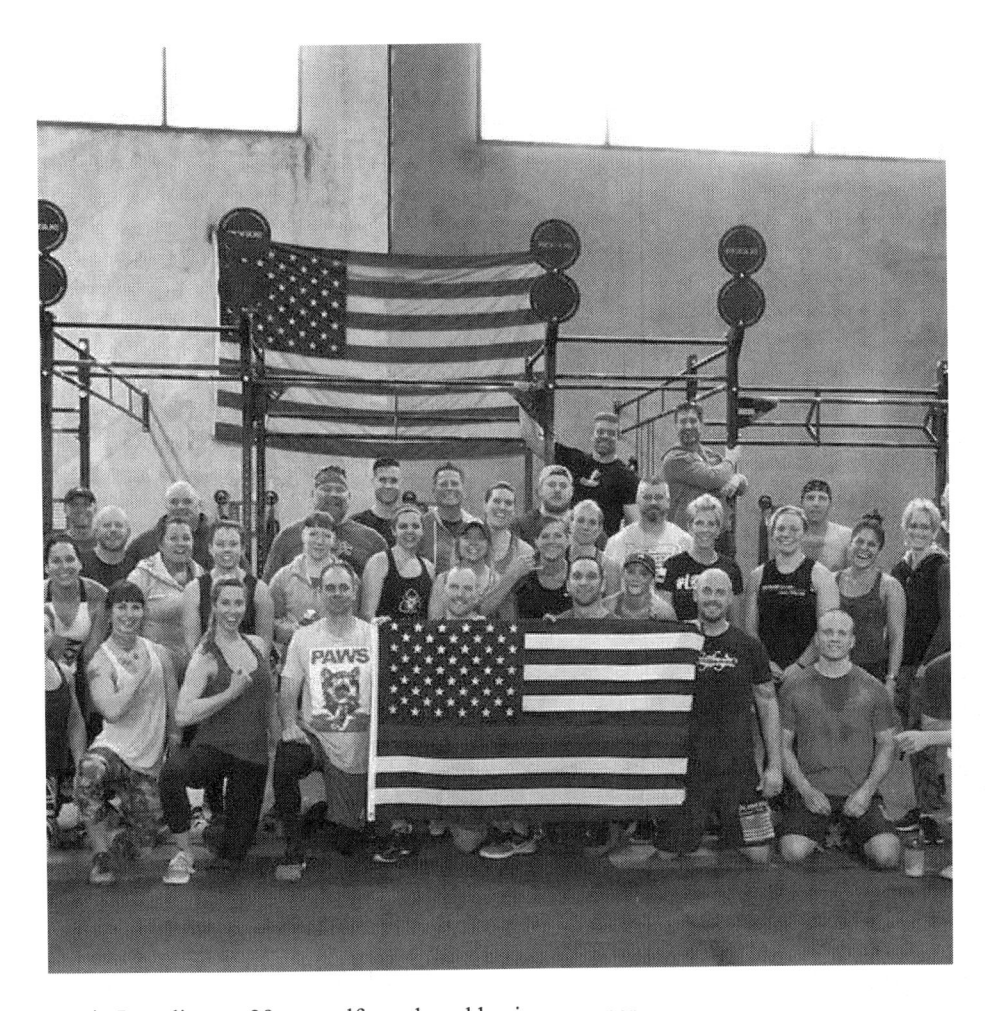

Kevin Iervolino   39   self-employed business owner

Kevin is a quiet, soft-spoken man who is built like a solid pro soccer mid-fielder. He comes to the 9 o'clock class and gets prepared early. When the workout is for partners, Kevin picks different people who will push him. He seems very self-sufficient and self-contained. He said that after high school he did little to keep fit. He would try things at home, but never found anything that could hold his interest.

He saw the Crossfit games on TV a few years back and it caught his attention. He stopped by CFOC and did some research on the internet and decided that he would probably enjoy the challenge of crossfit. He had recently been a kidney donor and that motivated him to get started.

Kevin is driven to get better. He wants to get pushed and to compete. He likes the challenge of crossfit and that it is a process – a long process – of continuing to improve. He says the community nature of CFOC is a bonus. He likes being around people who are building healthy habits for a lifetime. He loves the coaches and other members who will push him to do better in a workout or to learn a new skill.

He has a long view of crossfit. He believes that it takes time to build new habits and that it takes time to change fitness levels and to continue to improve. He has changed his nutrition and is looking at changing his workout schedule to provide new impetus for growth.

He says, "I love putting in the time. And I love the people." It makes me feel empowered to do everyday stuff well.

Kevin is one of the members I really admire. He was at my first workout and he is there for almost every workout. He does extra work on the skills he is trying to master, and he quietly does his best for every workout. There is no flash or attention seeking. He just shows up!

There are many members who "just show up." They are there every day. They do the workouts as well as they can for that day. They are not looking to be the fastest or the strongest in the box. They are looking to improve every day.

I have adopted that approach myself. I know it takes time. Being in a hurry does not speed things up. I look back to where I was a year ago and I am amazed at the progress I've made. I move differently. I hold myself differently. I feel so much better in so many ways. And I function better throughout the day. It is such a gift to be able to continue to grow in the company of others who are doing the same thing.

I get frustrated when I lose sight of the process. I want to be stronger now. I want my lifts to improve immediately. I want my posture to correct itself.

Then I remember that it takes a little bit every day, consistently. Day after day, workout out after workout. And the changes happen. Not overnight, but surely. As long as I do the work.

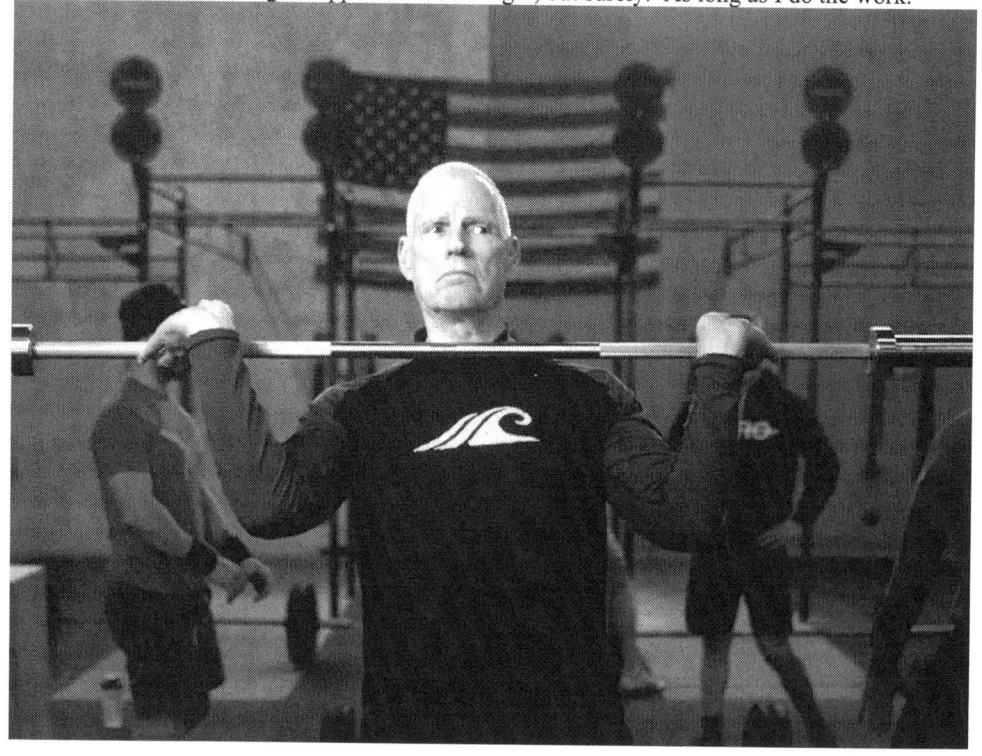

Today's workout was a doozy. Brad coached, so the box was open a half hour before the start. I got a good warmup while talking to a lot of folks who are not "usuals" for 9 AM. The "legends" were there – Hof, Tiny, and Don. There were also a bunch of the regulars, including Rachel and Gage, who I thought I would shadow for the workout. Instead, Tiny asked if I would like to partner and I jumped at the chance. Tiny is a large, friendly, bear of a man. He is hugely strong. He is a big personality. And he is an all-around great person.

The workout was a 35-minute metcon (metabolic conditioning) with a countdown rhythm. 50 cal row, 50 thrusters, 50 bar-facing burpees, and 50 pull ups. Then 40 of each, then 30 of each, then 20 of each, and finally 10 of each. It is a brutal scheme. I have never finished one of these in the time allowed. Both Tiny and I need to modify the workout to get the most out of it. I am doing dumbbell thrusters and burpees to a box, while Tiny is modifying the burpees and pull ups.

We kill the workout! It is so cool. We had a great pace on the rowing – I rowed faster than I ever have before. We kept moving throughout the whole workout – good pace, pushing to the limit and then a little more, and finished with 35 seconds left. I did not want to let Tiny down. It made for a great workout. We did not have the energy to do the shuttle runs with the extra time ☺

We got to hang out with "the guys" for a while after, talking golf and what we had planned for later. It was an amazing start to the day.

Then, I was able to talk with Brad for a bit about my goals for the rest of the year. He interrupted his workout to talk with me. He told me to go get my list, which I did, then we started going over my plan. For each item, Brad would walk over to the rack to show me a stretch or a movement. He showed me a couple of ways to work on my front rack position. He showed me some ways to work on mobility for the overhead lifts. He complimented me on having dates for completion on my goals and warned that I may not meet them all, but that I would make great progress. Then he also talked to me about nutrition and suggested that I talk with Jen about a new plan.

Brad is training for a competition in a month or so. I felt bad interrupting him. He was so gracious and helpful, giving me 20 minutes that he really didn't have. I love this place!

Todd A. Weber   50   Multnomah County Sheriff K-9 handler

Todd joined CFOC a few years after his wife, Liz. When I joined, we discovered the person who the DMV and others had been mixing up for years. Our names are spelled the same way. I was a K-9 handler in Viet Nam the year he was born. Scott is convinced that when we are in the same room, he can only see one or the other of us, not both. I call him my "ghost bro" as I am convinced that in another universe I died in Viet Nam and he was born to replace me.

Todd talks about how intense his first exposure to crossfit was. It was intimidating, challenging, and hard. He was used to working out at 24 HR Fitness and running on his own. He said he needed something more to stay in shape.

Not too long after he joined, he dislocated his shoulder on the job. He said that was when his loyalty to the box and to Jen and Scott was cemented. They worked with him every day to help with his recovery. They looked out for him and made accommodations whenever it was needed. Todd started working swing shift and could not attend any of the existing classes. Jen and Scott added a 10 o'clock class for Todd and others who wanted a less supervised class. A regular group of people, many of them in law enforcement, started working out at 10 with Todd.

He talks about how special the friendships are and how there is no worrying about cliques or not fitting in. You can be yourself. He said he has been humbled and gratified to be part of this community.

The Hero WODS help keep things in perspective for him. At the end of the day, he said, we are family.

During one pursuit on foot after a running suspect, Todd, his dog, and a SWAT team member were together. Todd said it was a long pursuit through trees and up and down hills. During one pause in the chase, the SWAT team member, who was much younger than Todd, said "For an old man you are in great shape!" Todd said to me, "That is real life crossfit."

Chapter Eight

The Ingredients

What is it that makes the CFOC or a Crossfit community so unique? What are the parts that create the feeling of "family?" Is it accidental or intentional? Does it require maintenance or is it self-sustaining?

Jen Cole Cereghino and Scott Cereghino 40,41   Owners, CFOC

Jen and Scott are an attractive young couple who are obviously very fit. Their passion and joy in what they do is magnetic. They complement each other in temperament and personality. They both laugh a lot.

Jen and Scott were active early in life. Jen did many different sports and got interested in nutrition and healthy eating due to a health concern. Scott was a basketball player who went on to play college basketball. They met in 2002.

Scott started doing cross fit in Richardson TX, where they settled. He was so sore the next day he had to go back. Jen was not interested. She asked Scott, "What about the cardio?"

Cross Fit had sectional competitions then and one was close to Richardson. Jen and Scott went to see the athletes compete. Jen said she saw two women competing and they were so amazing that she had to try it. She decided to give it one month, 4 days a week. She was totally intimidated. There were 3 or 4 people in her class, all guys. She loved the workouts!

She didn't want bulk, she wanted to compare her times as she progressed to see how she grew. She fell in love with it. She and Scott drew up a five-year plan to get back to Oregon and to start a box. Oregon City was the target. Scott was going to quit his job to move, when a competitor offered him a job based out of Portland. The timing was perfect.

Jen said that when they got to Oregon City, the Kreugers never stopped showing up to help`. She and Scott experimented with coaching, nutrition, and programming – working out of their garage. In August 2011 they got the warehouse space and started growing.

It was all word of mouth, Jen said. They modeled it after Cross Fit Richardson, where people could hang out before and after workouts. She said in Texas every day she looked forward to going to cross fit and she wanted the same feeling here. She and Scott talked a lot about being consistent with the focus on the needs of the members. They wanted the "family feel." They grew organically, friends hearing about it from friends.

Scott and Jen said that they wanted to have a place where the members could feel proud. The principles that guide them are:

    Cleanliness – equipment, space, restrooms all need to be extra clean.

    Respect – kids, parents, women, men - everyone will treat others with respect.

    Community – Scott and Jen will model the behavior they want to see in others. How Scott treats Jen, how Jen treats herself are standards for the community. They want the members to know that men and women can do anything they work for. They have a couple of sayings that they repeat often: "Mental confidence comes with competence" and "Let's get shit done."

    Calling out – it doesn't matter who you are if you work hard! Recognize the effort!

    Move well and move safely – No. 1 concern.

Jen is the first line of communication. She says she wants to work with the women members because many don't feel they deserve it or deserve the time it takes to get fit. She wants them to be an athlete again! She wants them to do something challenging! They can expect more of themselves. If you are working hard, you will change.

In programming the workouts, Jen's goal is for everyone to finish together.

The Hero workouts have special meaning for Jen and Scott. They feel members are more likely to push harder for a special workout. And the meaning helps us remember the sacrifice others have made.

For Jen and Scott, the "special sauce" is caring. Jen says that Becky Kreuger taught her how to do things without expecting anything in return and how to make people feel special. She says that she is still learning and growing.

Scott and Jen think that CFOC has great coaches. They all have full-time jobs and choose to coach because of their passion.

Jen says that for her, how people show up is the key. "As long as I can be part of this community, I will be OK!"

Both Jen and I were in tears at this point. Scott had left to work with a class. It was so moving to hear both Jen and Scott talk about the hopes they had for the box and how those hopes had translated into reality.

The community reflects Jen and Scott's values, modeling, and intentions. They walk their talk and encourage the rest of us to do the same. There is joy in the ability to conquer fear and gain mastery over physical movements that may have seemed impossible just a few months ago. There is satisfaction and pride in gaining control over what goes into your body and in shaping the muscles and movements. Being around people who are willing to do the work, who show up every day, who are positive and giving, who will sweat it out to the last rep, who support others with their whole hearts – this is special.

Chapter Nine

The Women of CFOC

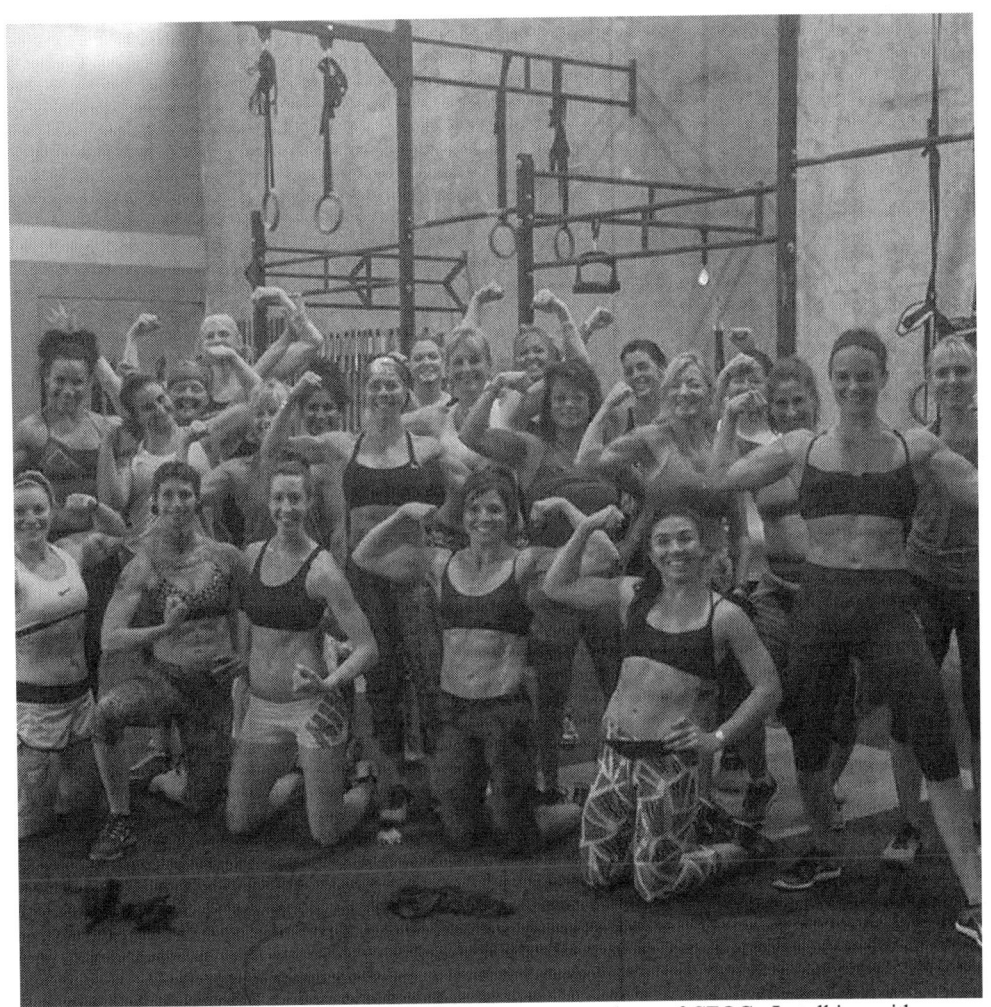

Jen talked about her goals for the women who become members of CFOC. In talking with her and Emily and the other women I was privileged to interview, I wanted to check on my observations to see if I was on track.

I believe that Jen has created a tribe of Warrior Women. Women who are confident, strong, self-aware, and self-assured. Women who have worked hard to gain the fitness they possess. Women who are comfortable in their bodies. Women who identify themselves as athletes.

Because of this, these women build each other up. They have no need to tear other women down or to belittle them. They support and help each other to grow and to work harder to become who they want to be. They treat other women differently and women treat them differently. There is a respect and admiration that is earned – and freely given.

In addition, they treat men differently and are treated differently by men. These women do not need affirmation and confirmation by others. They are secure in their sense of self. In a subtle, yet powerful way their equality is totally apparent. The relationships and connections with men are built on equal footing and a mutual respect and admiration.

There is no "locker room talk" among the men of CFOC. No one sexualizes conversations or objectifies women. We admire women's bodies because we know the amount of hard work and effort it takes to get there. There is a mutual understanding of the hard workouts endured, and the careful nutrition, and the lifestyle necessary to achieve these levels of fitness.

That is not to say that there is not playful banter and teasing exchanged. There is. But it never crosses the line into offensive or sexual language.

I asked Jen and Emily and other women about these observations to see if their perspective was the same. They said it was. And, they added, the women of CFOC have no need to bash men, as many feminists do. There is a connection in the effort, and sweat, and soreness, and mental toughness, and physical exhaustion of a good workout. Everyone suffers the same. Everyone celebrates. Everyone admires and recognizes the amount of work it takes. There are no differences.

Also, the shape of a woman's body does not have much bearing on how fit the person is. There are older women, younger women, thick women, flabby women, women recovering from diseases and injuries, women with kids and without. All are embraced without judgement or bias. All are athletes. And all are moving forward in creating a better person than yesterday.

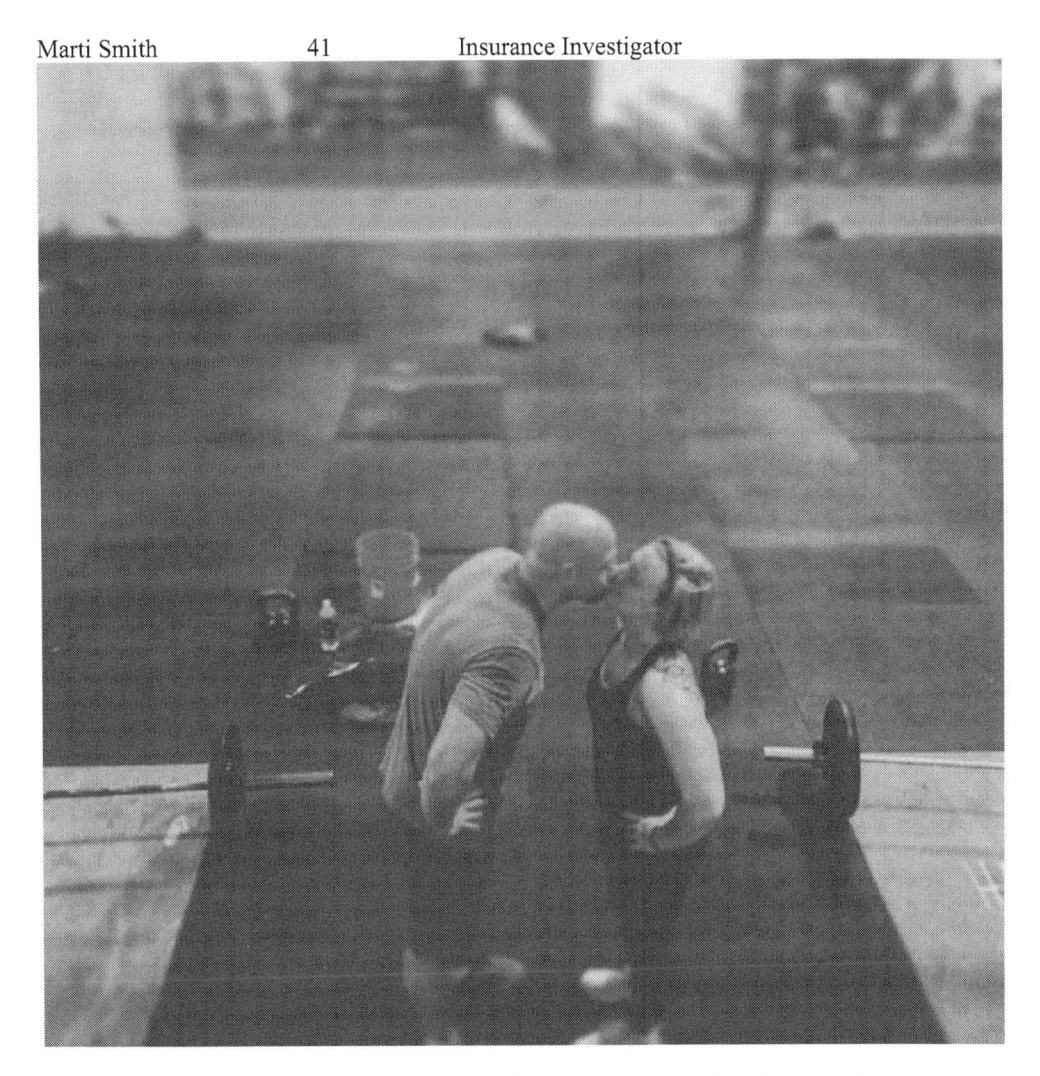

Marti is a strong woman. She has worked hard to get there. She played sports when she was younger – soccer and then dance team through high school. She started weightlifting in high school and really liked it. After high school she was not regularly active.

About 2005 she started working out again. She met her husband, Kyle soon after. He is a member of the Portland Police Bureau SWOT team and needed to stay in shape. He wanted to try cross fit and saw the window stickers for CFOC and gave it a try. He loved it!

They had a new baby and Marti was also working and she resented that Kyle had the time to do it and she didn't. He wanted her to join, but she didn't feel she could make the time.

She finally gave in. She was intimidated and introverted, so she came with a friend. She said that it was so tight knit – but everyone was so friendly and welcoming. At times she thought about going to a different gym, then she and Kyle started making close friends and it became family.

For Marti, there are two things that are amazing about CFOC. One is the support for other members. There was a house fire, and everyone helped the family. The cancer workouts and finding a wig for a woman who could not afford it also had an impact. Marti said that the CFOC family is more than just a family. It attracts the same kind of people – slightly obsessive and foxhole friends – fighting for each other. There is great mutual respect and admiration.

The second aspect of CFOC that stands out for Marti are the Hero Workouts. She comes from a military family and her husband is in law enforcement. This is my life, she said. It is so important to remember the men and women who sacrificed everything for us…and to support the families left behind.

Marti says that her confidence has grown so much since starting cross fit. She can own a room! And it doesn't stop there. The cross fit lifestyle creates huge changes in her whole life.

It is hard to describe the sense of calm strength and confidence that radiates from Marti. Like the other members of the tribe, she holds herself with a dignity that is obvious. She moves with power and grace. She is an athlete. And she can own a room.

Sue Stark　　　　62　　　　retired elementary PE teacher

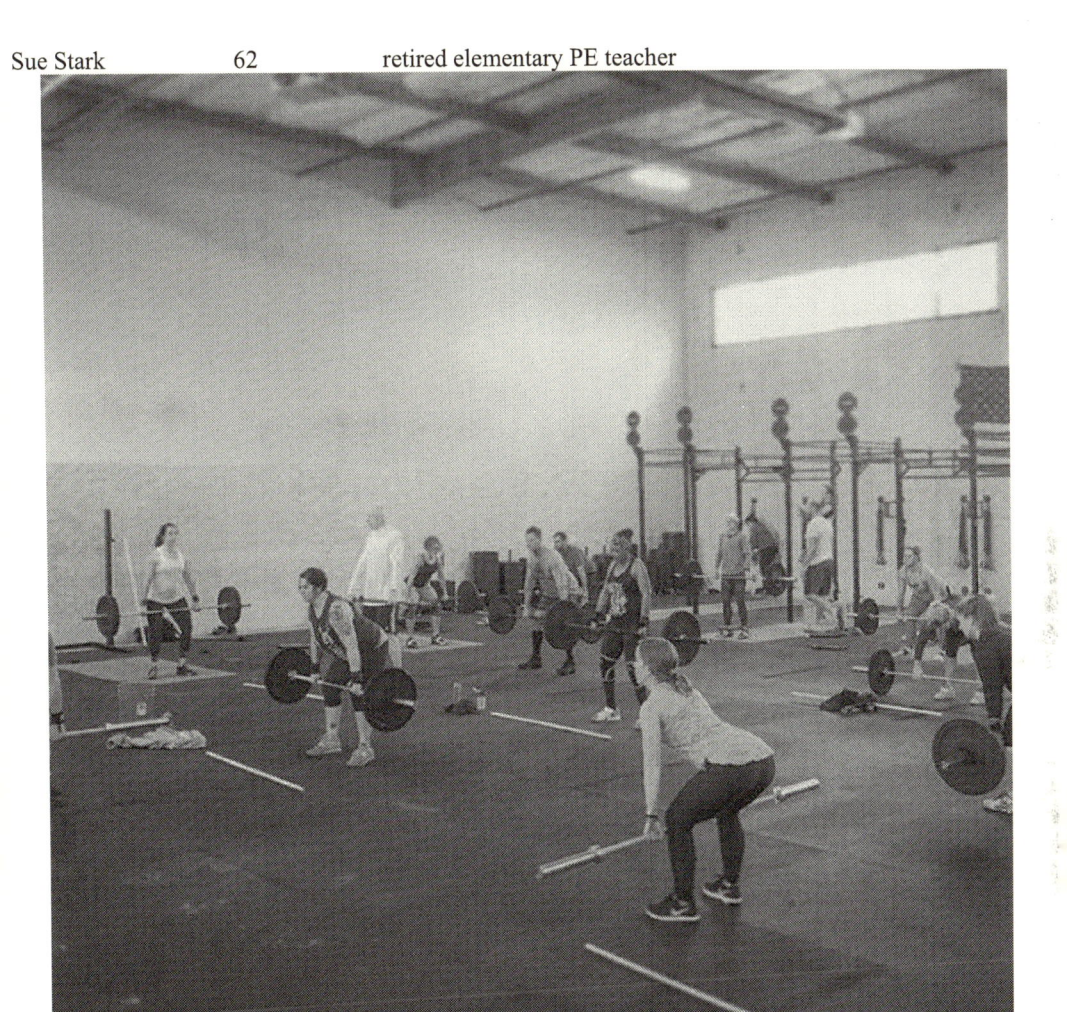

Sue is one of my workout buddies. She comes to the 9 AM class whenever she is not off doing retired things. She has an infectious energy and smile.

Sue has been active her whole life and wanted a place where she could stay fit and be around healthy people. She said she had been a member of a commercial gym in the past and did not like that the only person you really knew was the front desk person.

When you first join crossfit there is a lot of information to learn. Other members were very eager to help her learn and encouraged her as a new member. She resolved right then to make it a habit to always welcome new people and to make them feel comfortable when asking for help from other athletes. From my experience she has succeeded at that.

Her first partner WOD was a positive experience. She said that a young man ran over to her and asked if he could partner with her. She said it was a great workout.

Sue has a cancer project that is dear to her heart. She said that Jen and Scott heard about it and bought a whole table at a fund-raising event to support her and the project.

CFOC is like "Cheers," she told me. Everyone knows your name. She enjoys the special workouts as they remind her of how lucky she is. Her older sister died of a heart attack at 57 and Sue wants to remain a contributing member of the community for a long time.

Sue appreciates how educated the coaches are. And she loves Jen for her attitude of compassion.

Today's workout was another killer. I missed yesterday playing golf, so I was ready to go hard. I partnered with Natalie and it was great. We did a run, then dumbbell snatch, then run, then dumbbell snatch, then 1 rep max clean and jerk. I got a PR for the clean and jerk– 100#s. Then it was 15 minutes of 20 burpees to box step overs with weight and 25 pull ups per round AMRAP. Natalie and I completed 3 rounds and 15 reps, and it was hard – sweaty, sweaty hard! It felt so good to be done. What a great way to start the weekend.

Ashley Rios — 34 — mortgage lender

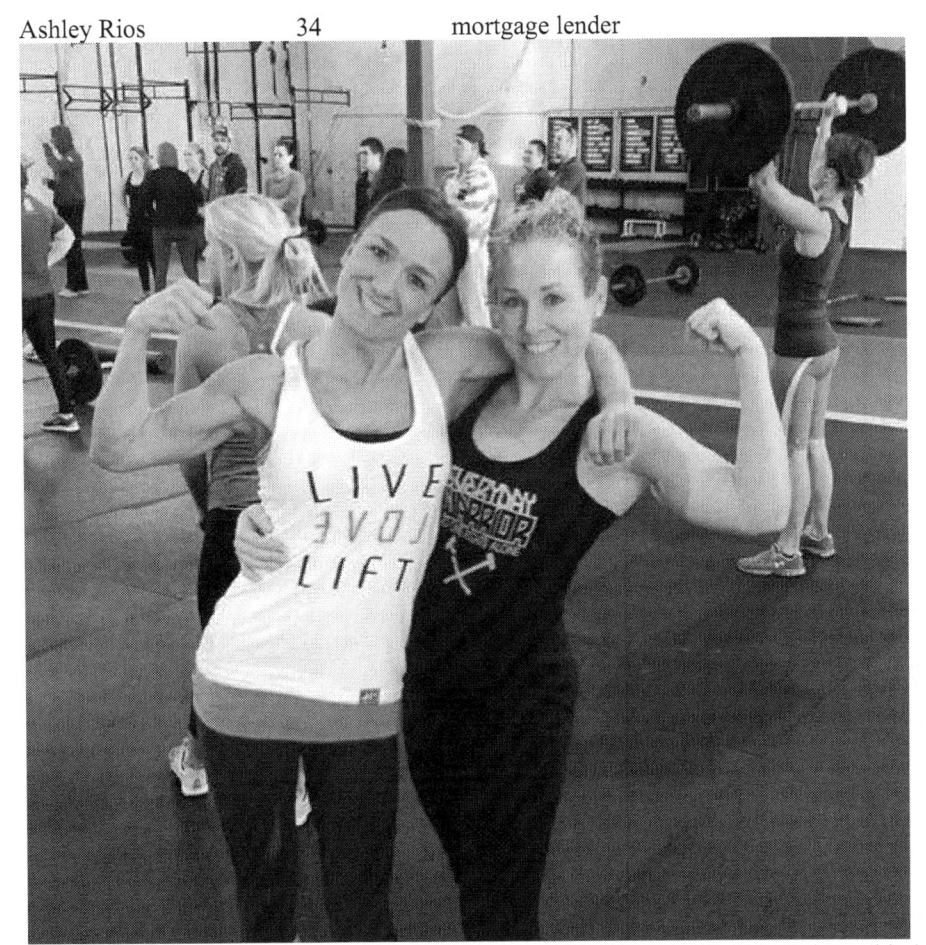

Ashley has a background as a competitive athlete. She played softball and cheered in high school. She stopped being active during her pregnancies and then wanted to give crossfit a try. She tried several boxes but did not like that the coaches lacked basic knowledge of fitness and that the boxes were not close knit as a community.

She met Jen and Scott and liked their focus on health and form and their obvious passion, knowledge and how they looked out for people. She tried CFOC for a couple of weeks and really liked the differences from the other boxes. She said that she felt that Jen and Scott care about the members. And, she said, if they are pushing themselves this hard, so can I.

Here are her reasons for being a member of CFOC and a member of the tribe for 4 years:
- The owners have passion and go out of their way to give individual care
  - Jen "notices" how you are doing. She is "dialed in" and respects where you are as an athlete
  - Jen is a "mother figure" who has taught her how to feel good about herself and how to let go of the impact of things outside the box

She loves that all the coaches are engaged and passionate

She loves being in this environment. She can be vulnerable, having a mental battle, pushing through, and Jen may say that "today is just not the day"

Ashley says that it is always challenging, always different, and that her awareness builds after each workout.

CFOC is unlike any other place! No matter who you are, you can do crossfit.

The themes are the same with most members: warm, inviting, challenging, engaged and passionate. That is CFOC and Crossfit. And, a big piece of those feelings is generated by the members themselves.

For older athletes, the atmosphere of acceptance and no judgement is crucial. It allows us to be vulnerable again and to accept the help that is offered. My first workouts were intimidating and scary. But there was always someone there to offer help and guidance and to encourage me. It was incredible.

Once I realized that I was not supposed to know what I was doing and that part of the process is leaving the ego at the door, I was able to relax into the role of a beginner. And, I still am! I feel like a kid again. I am learning new things. I am playing with my friends. I am gaining confidence in new movements. I am struggling to master new things. It is so much fun!

Chapter Ten

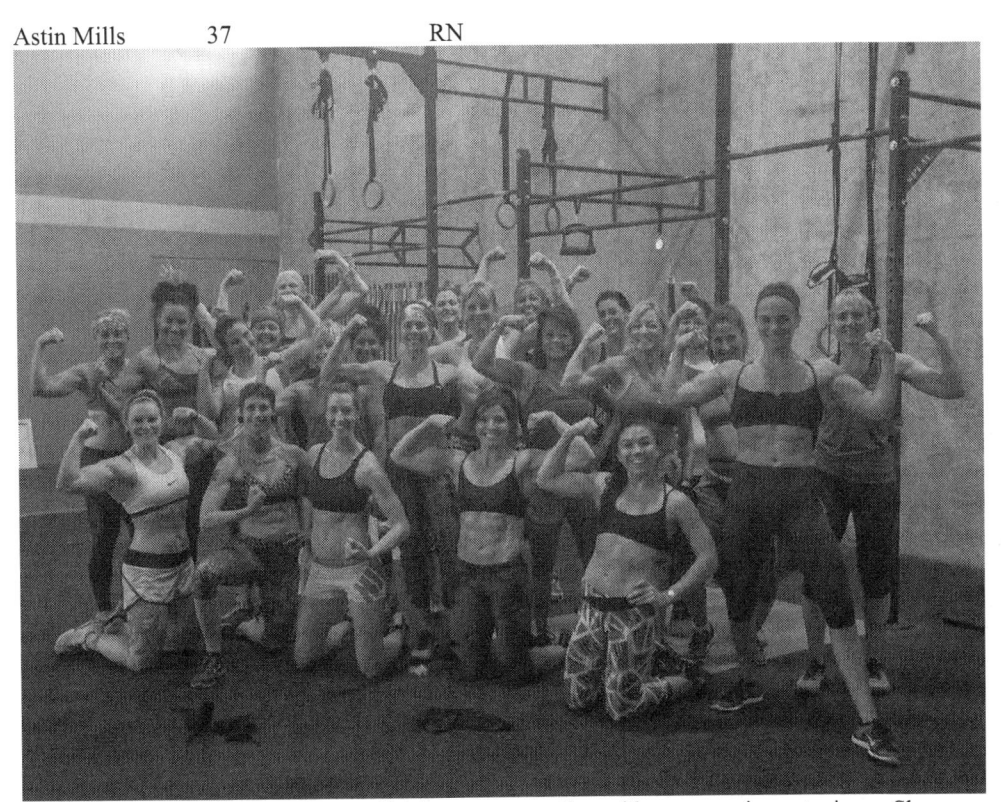

Astin Mills   37   RN

Astin is a special lady in my heart. She has a great smile and her energy is contagious. She grew up a tomboy in Alaska and was involved in many sports. After a stint in the air force as a nurse, she and her family moved to Oregon City. She said that she was pretty inactive for six years. Then 3 years ago, she decided to investigate crossfit. She decided on CFOC because she could bring her kids and that it felt warm and secure.

She is in the 9 AM class most of the time. She said that she felt like a stranger in the afternoon classes. She said that she tried to reach out to others – to step outside her comfort zones.

When I had been going to the 9 AM class for about 6 or 7 weeks, Astin walked over to sit by me after a workout. She said she was Astin. I replied that I knew, and I was Todd. Then the most remarkable thing happened. She said, I am going to be your friend. We are going to work out together and get to know each other and that we would always have each other to talk to.

I was totally blown away. I had never had someone reach out so warmly and with an open heart to be my friend. She was true to her word. We worked out together, talked a lot, laughed a lot, and became friends. I love Astin so much. Whenever I see her, it makes my day. I will be forever grateful to her.

Astin said that she became spellbound by the competitive opportunities and decided to participate in the summer games. She said that she and her partner did the best that they could, everybody celebrated, that it was so motivating. She wants to be "the best I can be" – not to beat others, but to better herself.

She says that CFOC is safe and emotionally validating. It is exciting to be around – it is family – an amazing community that pulls you along. "Show up as you are!" she says. The workouts destroy everything and then build it back up.

Astin wrote back to me after I showed her a draft: I so appreciate the kind words you wrote about me. I have a sentiment that I don't know if it was adequately shared when we interviewed - it's the kind of 'self-discovering' that has taken years to work out for myself and who knows how clearly I described it, or even if I tried to (I can't remember now). There was a period of time when I felt intimidated and insecure as I showed up for classes - that "I don't know anybody and so I'm alone and the odd man out" feeling. I made a decision to reach out and take the first step in connecting with others - I can't complain about nobody talking to me if I haven't first tried to reach out first. Connecting with you...and also Meighan...were examples of that effort I decided to make - I made an active decision to put my insecurity on a shelf for a bit and just reach out. It's amazing how many doors that has opened for me, and it completely changed my perception of the community at the gym.

Today's workout was a killer! Jen is programming for the Best in the West games, and the workouts have some extra zest.

Today we do 3 10-minute linked segments with a partner. The first segment is a 10 cal row and then max alternate dumbbell snatches. Partners switch every 1 minute – one on and one off. Then without pause, the second segment is 15 wall balls, then max ab-mat sit ups. Switching every minute. The last segment is 10 thrusters, then max lateral burpees. The pace is to go all out if possible. My goodness!

Adam asked me to partner and I went for it. Adam has been around for about 7 or 8 months now and he is a total maniac. He goes full steam, all out, all the time. For a while he was doing two workouts a day until Jen told him to cool it. He is 47 or 48, probably OCD, and a wild man. He is a Trump supporter and I wear protest t-shirts. We get along really well though.

He probably goes all in at work, at gambling, at drinking and anything else he tries. When he first started, I would partner with him often, and then he got too strong and too fast. One of the Tylers said that Adam wants to have 4 yrs' cross fit experience in one year. It came as a surprise that he asked me to partner. I did not want to slow him down.

We went crazy – or at least Adam did. We beat the best score for the day – so far. That made Adam happy. I was just happy to catch my breath again.

Today is Thursday – rest day and mobility and flexibility. I am working on the suggestions that Brad gave me last week and on the muscle imbalance that is part of my continuing struggle. It means I need to get stronger on my left side and to work on the stabilizer muscles all up and down that side.

 I start with the stretches that Brad gave me for my chest, triceps, and wrists to help with the front rack position. My wrists need a lot of work so I can get my elbows up in the proper position.

 While I am working on this, Tiny and Hof come in to do some work. Tiny has his son, Henry, with him. He is a ball of energy. We start talking and decide to play golf on Monday. They are both coming to the 9 AM class tomorrow and Tiny wants to partner again. Cool!

 I go to work on my balance and strength on my left hip and leg. It is surprisingly hard. All those little muscles quiver and shake. It's going to be a long process and I'm ready to make it happen.

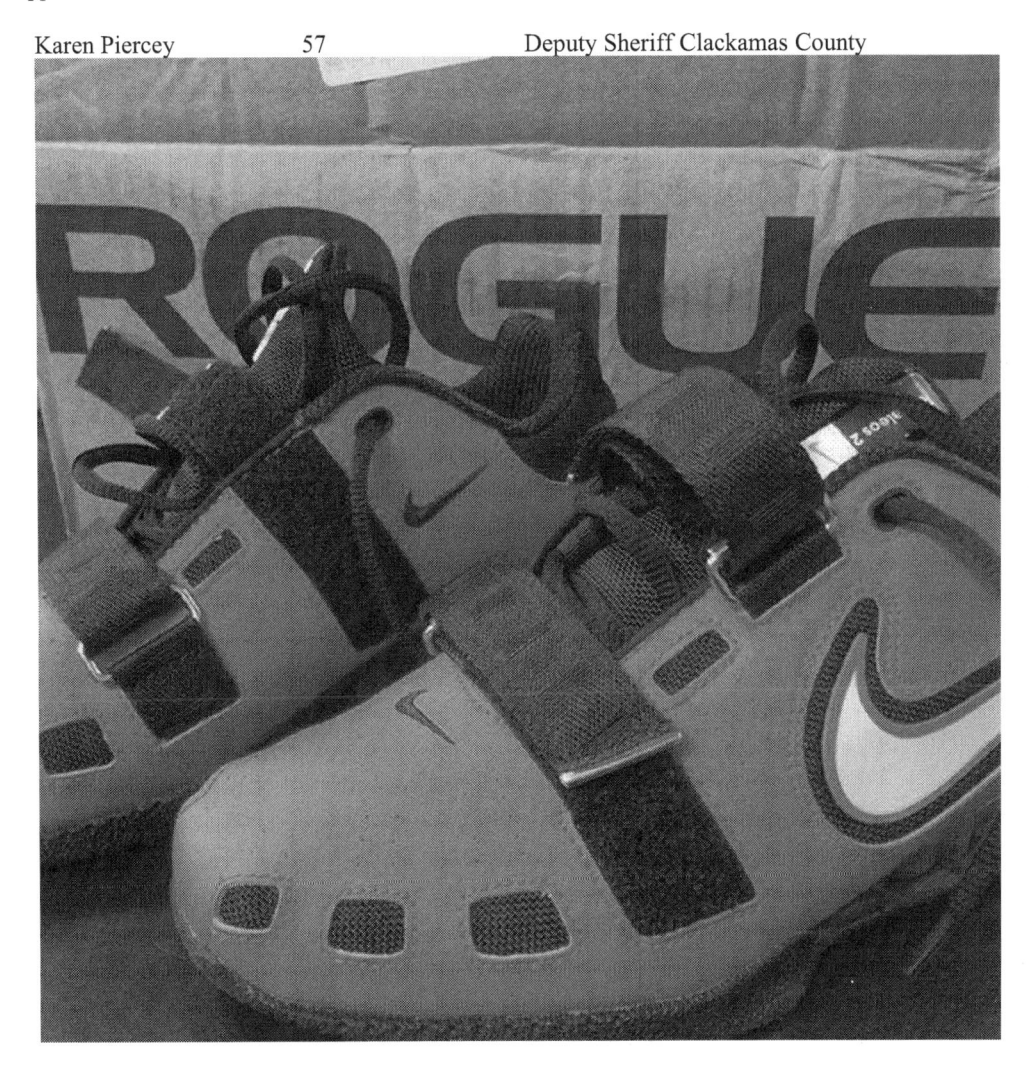

Karen Piercey   57   Deputy Sheriff Clackamas County

Karen is a powerful woman. She needs to be for her job in the County Jail. She went into the army after high school and was in tip top shape. She was in a car accident in 1995 which resulted in a bad neck. She let her physical condition go, gained weight, and smoked.

Finally, she had enough and started looking for a place to get back into good shape. She thought that crossfit was for "knuckle draggers" and didn't think she would be interested. As she went back and forth to work, she would see people running in the parking lot, saw the sign for CFOC, and walked in. She said that she knew right away that "this is a good gym." She felt right at home.

Yes, cross fit is different. She discovered that she had not been lifting properly. Several of the coaches helped her determine what she wanted to accomplish. She said that she is here to get better. That she needs to be patient. No one here is judgmental. They genuinely care. Everyone enjoys and loves what they are doing and want to help each other meet their goals.

She said that she has a sense of family every time she comes to CFOC. Everyone helps and encourages. People root for you. I feel so fortunate to belong to this gym, Karen says. There is nothing like a good sweaty hug! I never want to stop – it is life changing.

She says that she didn't realize that women could be this strong. She feels stronger now than she ever has. She knows she will never totally arrive. It has impacted every aspect of her life.

For the aging athlete, this sense of family, of belonging, is crucial to good health. There is a lot of research that confirms that feeling connected leads to well-being. It is part of the concept of "fitness" that I am proposing in this book.

If we push our bodies with intense exercise every day we move toward fitness. If we eat good, whole foods with lots of green leafy vegetables, we move toward fitness. If we get a good night's rest every night, we move toward fitness. And, if we are connected, a part of something bigger than we are, a place where we belong, we move toward fitness.

All of this together impacts aging. It slows down the process. It creates healthier cells. It increases muscle mass and bone density. It helps improve balance and coordination. It improves our sense of well-being. It fights depression. It cuts down the risk of age-related chronic diseases. It can increase our quality of life for a long time.

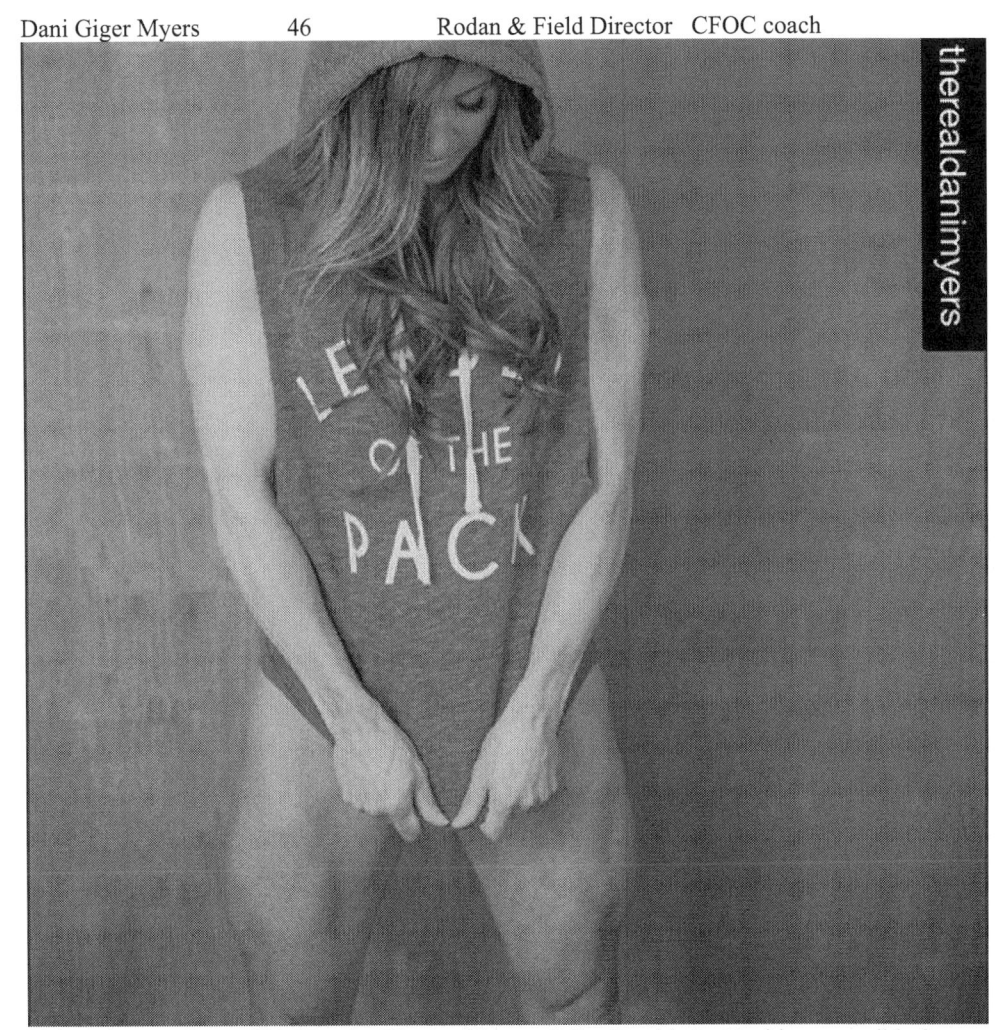

Dani Giger Myers   46   Rodan & Field Director   CFOC coach

therealdanimyers

If there is an assistant Chief for the Warrior Women Tribe, Dani is it. Dani is responsible for recommending CFOC to many, many people. She is a beast when it comes to fitness. And she is Jen's partner for competitions.

Dani did cheer in high school then decided to take up body building and powerlifting. She worked for a Nautilus gym for quite a while and managed to have four children while maintaining an incredible fitness level.

She started crossfit a couple of years after Steve and Karla Martin suggested it. She said it was mainly to get out of the house after baby number 4. She started working out at the box. She became a dedicated crossfit athlete.

With her background, she became an excellent coach at the box. Dani has been a personal trainer for 25 years and has a Bachelor of Science in Exercise and Sport Science from Oregon State University. She started coaching at CFOC after almost 5 years of being a crossfit athlete. Her deep understanding of anatomy and physiology as well as movement provides a wonderful base for helping the members.

She can spot a small hitch or issue with a movement; help you figure it out and "feel" it and then give you a way to correct it. She does it in such a way that you feel that you figured it out for yourself. She is a great coach.

She sets a great example in the box for other women (and men) to follow. She works hard in her workouts and attacks weaknesses with gusto.

Another whopper of a workout today. My goodness. I think that my humility is at an all-time high (low?) from this week's workouts.

Today was brutal. It started with weight work. I chose to do weighted sled pulls – 400#s times 7 every two minutes. My legs were shaking so hard!

Then we did a twenty-minute AMRAP of 20 cal row, 20 Kettle bell swings, and 20 weighted step ups. After the sled pulls, my legs were toast doing the rows, swings and step ups. I am not sure that I have ever sweated this much during a workout. And I feel like I am totally out of shape to do this kind of workout. I was glad to hear that other people felt the same way and it wasn't just me.

It took about 5 minutes to cool down from the workout and then people started talking about who would be here tomorrow. That's cross fit.

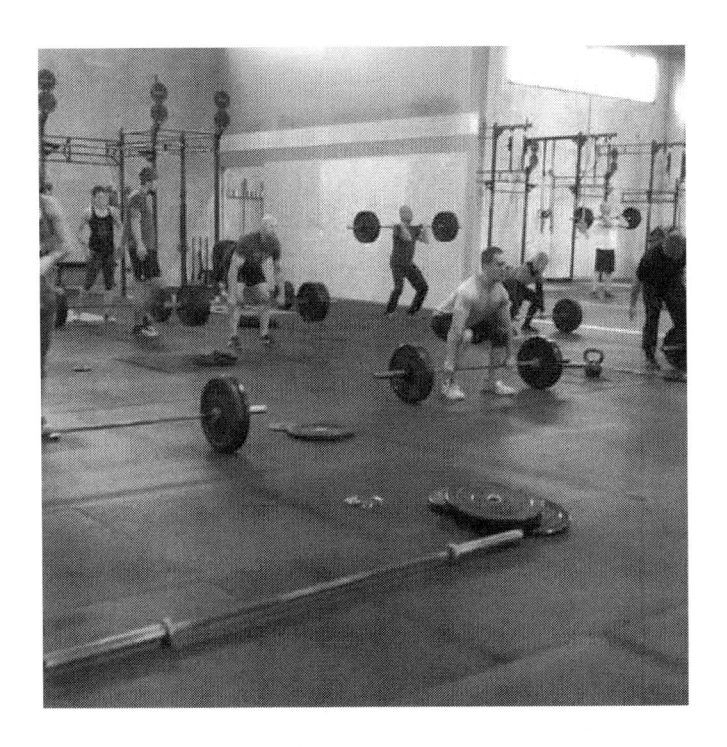

It has been hot lately. More people are showing up for the 9 AM workouts to avoid the afternoon heat. It has been a bit crowded and more fun with the energy in the box.

Yesterday and today we did individual workouts with some tough components. Today's workout is a repeat from last month. We will use it to check our progress.

It consists of 6 rounds of 3 minutes on and 3 minutes off. For me, it is a 200m run, followed by 5 deadlifts and max burpees to a box. I am working on my form for the deadlifts – getting my back flat and shoulders back – so I am lifting from 6" boxes. It was 8" last time so I am making good progress.

Even though it is 9 AM, it is hot outside, and I am soaking in sweat by the end of the first round. It is a fun – though very tough – workout with a good group of people. I really pushed it and felt super once I catch my breath. I do some extra work on my core because this week I've been feeling all the activation while doing the workouts. That is really good, because in the past I would not remember to activate my core and I would let power leak from my body. The things you learn doing cross fit... It is amazing. Also, Dani gave me a great tip about my elbows doing deadlifts. It really helped.

Kori Mehdikhan   30 yrs old   Kari Hansen   CPA/PR

Kori was a competitive athlete in high school playing soccer and competitive cheerleading. She was also a runner. After two years in college, she quit working out and gained a bunch of weight.

After working in Eugene for 4 years, she found CFOC. It was intimidating at first, but people were so friendly she said that it was easy to stay involved. After being at the box for one month she met Kari Hansen, who is still her workout partner.

They both talk about how meeting their best friend and being able to compete together, being part of a group together, having similar goals, and bonding over the journey they share – it makes it so special!

They both said that it is really difficult to put words to the experience – suffering together, wanting to get better, having someone to share it all with. It is incredibly special.

Kari said that it is like watching the big kids on the playground. "I want to do that!" It is fun and challenging. Starting is hard, but it is more than worth it.

Both Kari and Kori own their bodies in such a way that it is clear they don't need your approval or permission to be and do who and what they please. If I had daughters and granddaughters, I would want them to be members of their tribe.

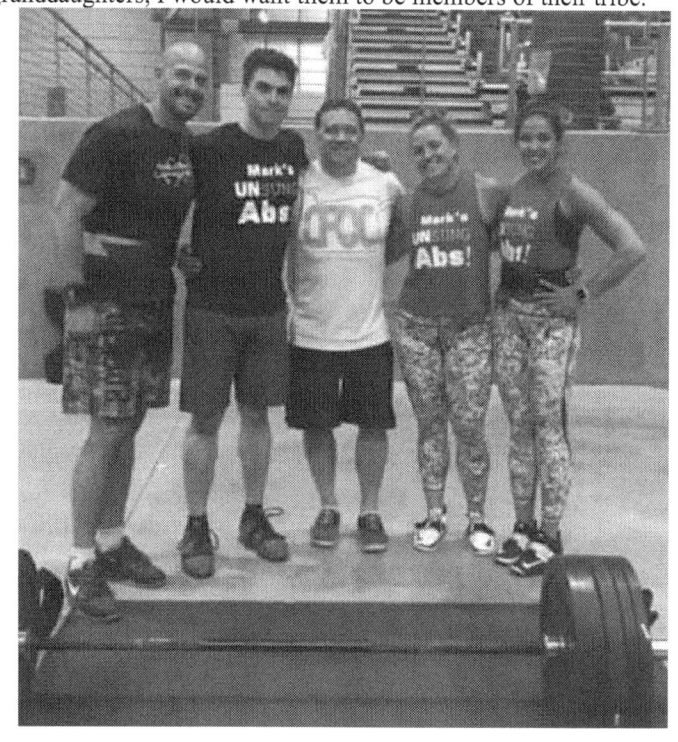

Leilani Lopes 20 years old   pre-med student PSU

Leilani is a native of crossfit land, not an immigrant. She started working out with her father, Kelii, at home when she was 7. She played club soccer and other sports, then started at CFOC when she was 12.

She says she was a little small for the equipment and was obviously the youngest, but everyone was positive, accepting and welcoming. She said there was some kind of force that encouraged working hard and she enjoyed it. She dislocated her knee and could no longer play soccer and she missed the competition, so she put her energy into crossfit.

She and her dad used Invictus programming and she decided she wanted to compete in the crossfit games. She says she has a lot of things to fix if she wants to compete at the highest level.

She loves the community and says she has gained so much from crossfit:
- It is character building.
- It is supportive and empowering.
- She doesn't need to meet the image society wants.
- It is a totally level playing field.
- Everyone has a goal and holds each other accountable.

Leilani is a compact, powerful athlete. She is striking in her ease and grace and strength. She is an inspiration to me.

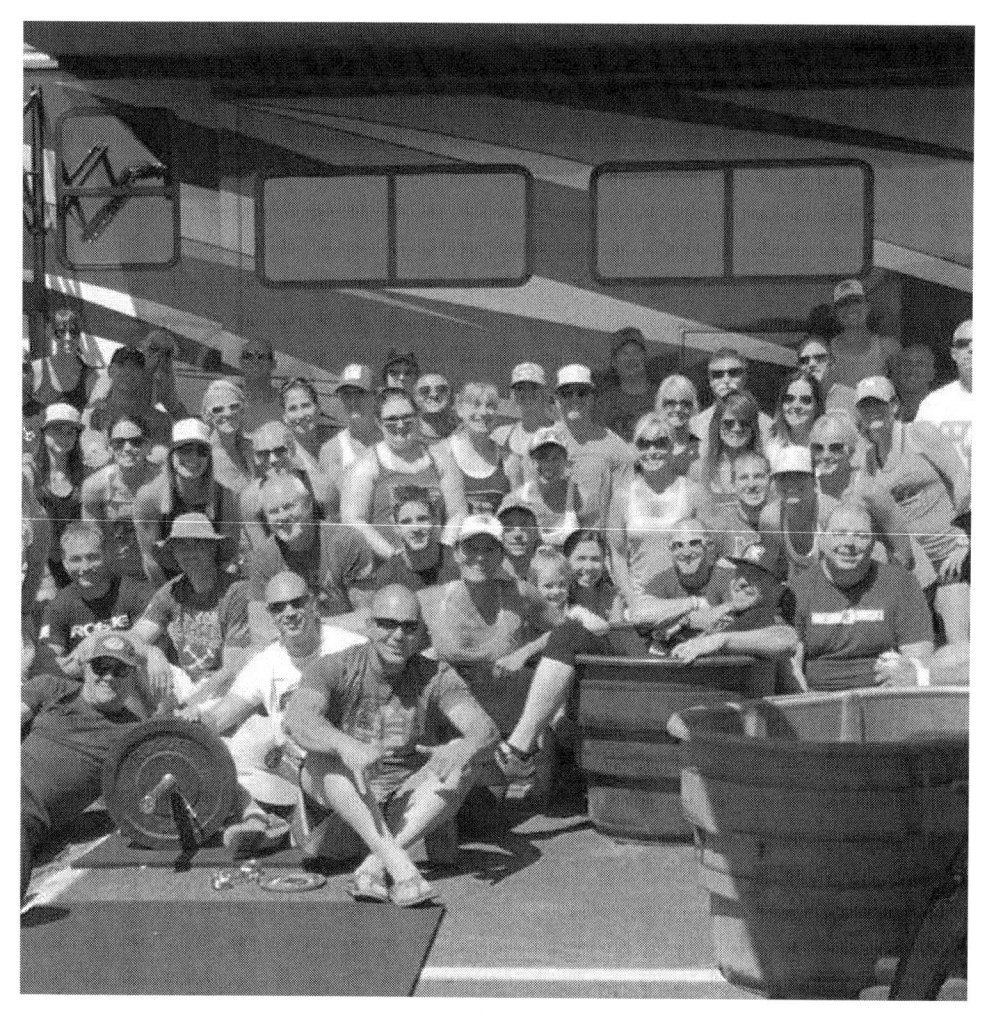

Cross fit can be a cause for contemplation and soul-searching. Why am I putting in this much effort and time for my fitness? Is it appearance? Is it functionality as I age? Is it to be capable of doing my job? Is it to remain active with my family and friends?

As I mentioned earlier, CFOC members are doers. They make things happen. They contribute to the greater good – in whatever way makes sense for them. I think crossfit fosters this kind of motivation. We want to make a difference. We want to be capable of doing the work to make that happen. I think crossfit goes hand in hand with personal health, community health, and being part of something greater than ourselves.

We'll explore some of the aspects of CFOC's involvement in giving in the next section.

Chapter Eleven

Giving Back
Hero WODS, Special WODS, and Community Support WODS

CFOC places special emphasis on doing workouts that support, celebrate and/or remember those who need our help, those who have sacrificed to protect us, and those who marking a special day. It is our way of demonstrating our solidarity with our community.

Today's WOD is an example of that. It is the 7th Anniversary of CFOC's opening this week, and there is a workout today and one on Saturday to celebrate the event.

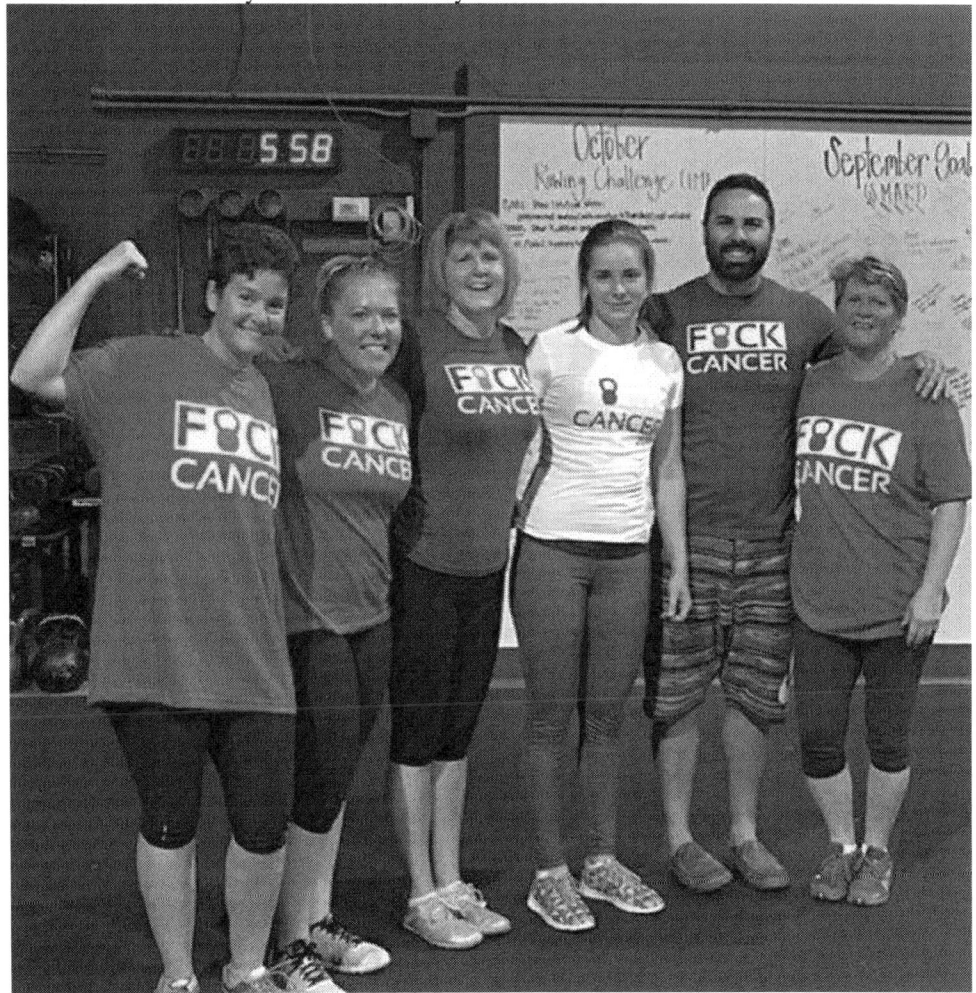

Today is a partner WOD built around the date of the opening. Sue and I do this work out together. It starts with 8 rounds of 8 shoulder to overhead lifts and 18 abmat sit-ups. Then we do 175 m of bear crawls/dance moves. Then comes a 2011m row. Then another 175 m of bear crawls or dance moves. And it finishes with 8 rounds of 8 weighted step overs and 11 kettle bell swings. Sue and I have a great time doing this together. On the bear crawls we do about half bear crawls and half dance moves. I am getting my groove thing on and having a great time. We finish the workout in 32 minutes, and I am dripping in sweat. It is so much fun. That is the purpose of these kinds of workouts… To celebrate and/or to remember and/or to support.

We do celebration workouts for member birthdays (the big ones), and for special occasions. We celebrate the holidays with special workouts. The holiday workouts tend to be huge. It is so much fun working out with people you don't get to see that often and to get caught up with new members, folks coming back from being gone for a while, and folks whose regular classes don't match up with your schedule. The is always lots of laughter and energy.

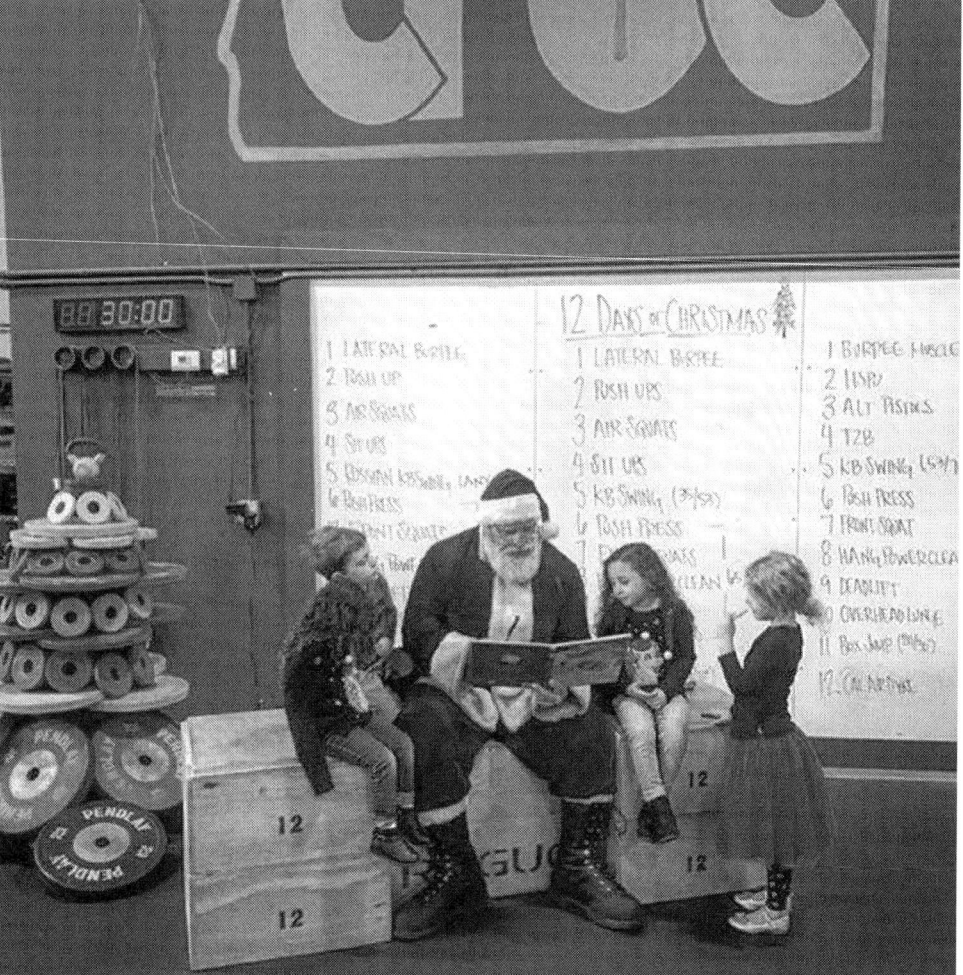

At Christmas, the box also supports local families who are going through a rough patch. Members organize tags that show a gift that each family needs and members take a tag or two or more and buy the gift, bring it back to the box with the tag, and it is distributed to the families right before Christmas. The tag could be for a gift card to the local grocery or for a winter coat for a 10 yr old boy, or for a toy for a 4 yr old. Last year we supported 4 families and it was super!

The Hero Workouts are different.

Probably the best-known Hero Workout is "Murph." Michael Patrick Murphy was a Navy Seal who won the Medal of Honor for his actions under fire during the War in Afghanistan. I don't know if the workout started with crossfit, but it has become a tradition in many different organizations.

The workout is done over Memorial Day Weekend at most boxes. It consists of a 1-mile run, then 100 pull ups, 200 pushups, 300 squats, and a 1-mile run. It seems simple – and it is. But it is brutal. The purpose for CFOC is to remember and show respect for a hero (and others) who made the ultimate sacrifice to protect our country. It is about symbolically showing the will and discipline to go the extra "mile" – the extra rep, the extra minute – in honor of those who gave it all. It is about pushing yourself beyond your limits. It is about remembering that if they can make that kind of sacrifice, we can give a little bit more ourselves.

We have a former Navy Seal as a member of CFOC and he gives a little talk before the start of "Murph" to remind us what making this kind of sacrifice means and to urge us to show the respect that Murph deserves.

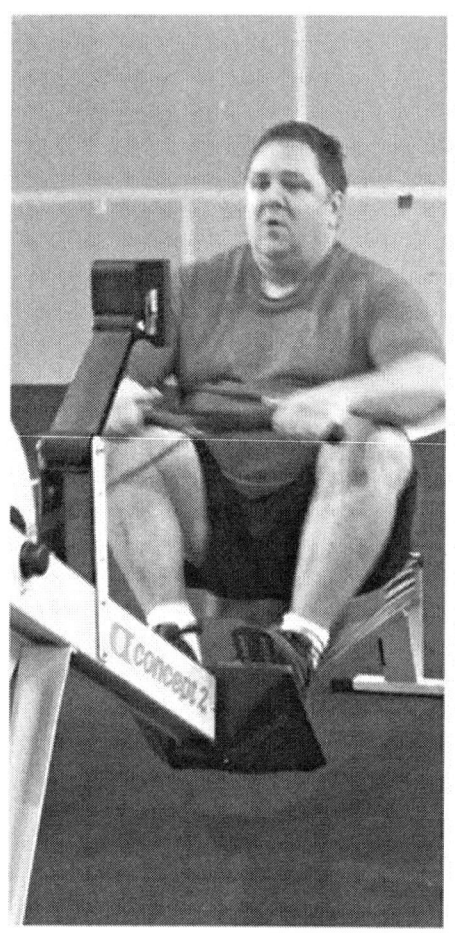

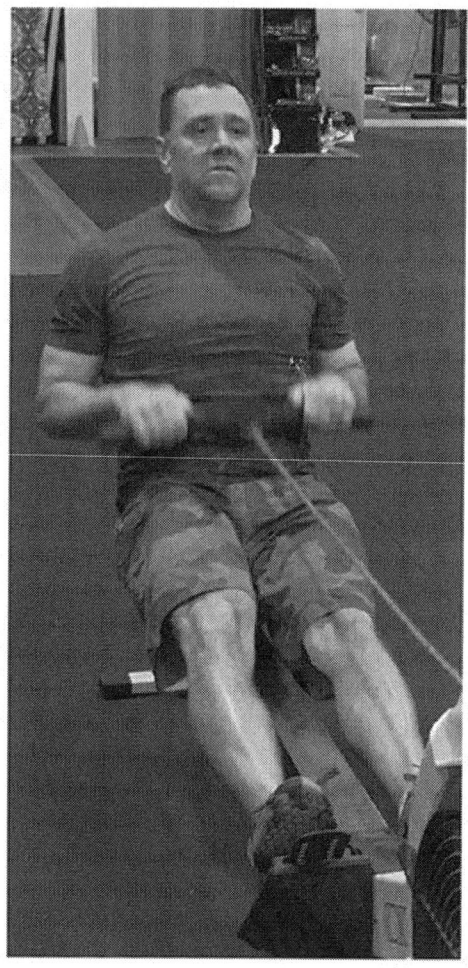

Mark MacDonald   49   sales/marketing manager CFOC coach

Mark grew up an excellent athlete. In high school he played soccer, baseball, and ran. He got inspired by the movie "Chariots of Fire" and switched to cross country running for his last years in high school. He would do extreme workouts at 4 AM to prepare for the season.

He entered The Citadel for college and continued to run. He had a great experience at The Citadel and probably would have graduated and gone into the Army. However, he had a falling out with his dad, left school and joined the Navy to become a Seal.

He joined the Navy in 1987 and joined Seal Team 8 in 1988. He was operationally deployed 7 times. His specialty was communications.

He left the Navy in 2000 and kicked around for a bit before marrying his wife, who he met in the Service. He started working in the defense industry and became a successful marketing and sales manager. He slowly stopped working out and over time went from about 200 #s to 310#s in 2010. He was morbidly obese.

He was in the ER every 4 months or so, it was difficult to do everyday things, and in 2012 he became extremely sick. His wife thought that crossfit might help. He met Abe and Steve, and then Jen and Scott and he signed up. The first year he lost 45 #s. He was still boozing. He wanted to quit crossfit. He was complaining about everything. Jen and Scott told him to "Just show the f#%* up" and Jen taught him how to perimeter shop (stay out of the interior aisles of the grocery store). He lost another 55 #s over the next year.

He went to his physician for a checkup and he was told, "Whatever you are doing, just keep doing it!" He lost a total of 140 #s. He says he is the healthiest he has been since being a teenager. He says that it transfers into every part of his life.

Mark got his Level One Certification and is a coach for CFOC. He believes that Jen saved his life. He does say that you can't help someone who does not want to help themselves, however.

He says that crossfit is not a panacea. If you like it, do it! In that case, it is the answer. He says that crossfit prepares you to be a jack of all things – master of none. He thinks the Olympic lifting is the most beneficial. It is the most criticized. He says the reality is that we are trained correctly in crossfit.

Jen and Scott set the tone. You get back what you put in. It is family.

He feels healthy and more confident. His goal is to do stuff. Food is how we look – fitness is how we feel. This is the place to be.

Mark is an inspiration and reminder for the box. He walks his talk. He offers admiration and respect. He is quick to greet new people and to recognize their efforts in making changes. He lets you know that he sees you working out and appreciates what you are doing. He is a good man.

I know that Mark is not the only one who hugely appreciates the Hero WODs. There are many veterans among the members of CFOC as well as law enforcement folks and fire fighters. All these people deserve recognition and respect and the Hero workouts are a way of showing that.

I told Marti Smith's story in The Women of CFOC section. There was one part I left out. As I said, she comes from a family with a military tradition and her husband is in law enforcement.

Marti told me a story about her husband and crossfit that is amazing. One night when Portland was in the grip of one of its infamous ice storms, her husband Kyle was assigned to traffic duty to help with the tangled traffic. He was on a high freeway overpass where a car had spun out on the black ice and smashed into the railing. Kyle was out of his car to set flares when a Ford Taurus came around the bend too fast and started sliding directly at Kyle.

Kyle told Marti that he only had a second to make a choice of what to do. He could go over the railing to certain serious injury or death or he could use crossfit. He did a box jump over the hood of the sliding car, just catching his foot on the driver's side mirror, which set him tumbling. Nothing was broken. Before crossfit, Kyle was overweight and out of shape. Marti says that thanks to crossfit he is alive today.

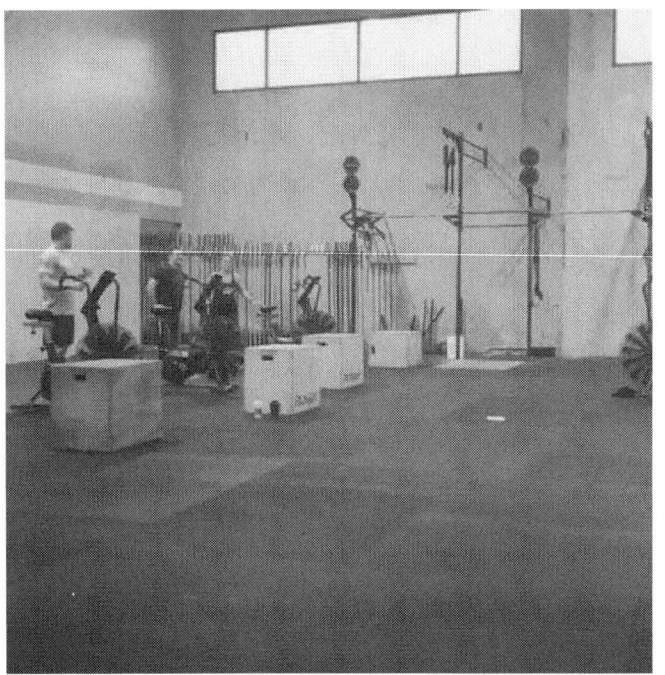

Those are the kinds of experiences that make the Hero WODs so important. They are not just a "memorial," but are a living testament to grit and perseverance and continuing to strive when it seems there is nothing left but will power and discipline.

There are other heroes who are celebrated and supported at CFOC. These are the members and others who are fighting a battle with cancer and other debilitating diseases.

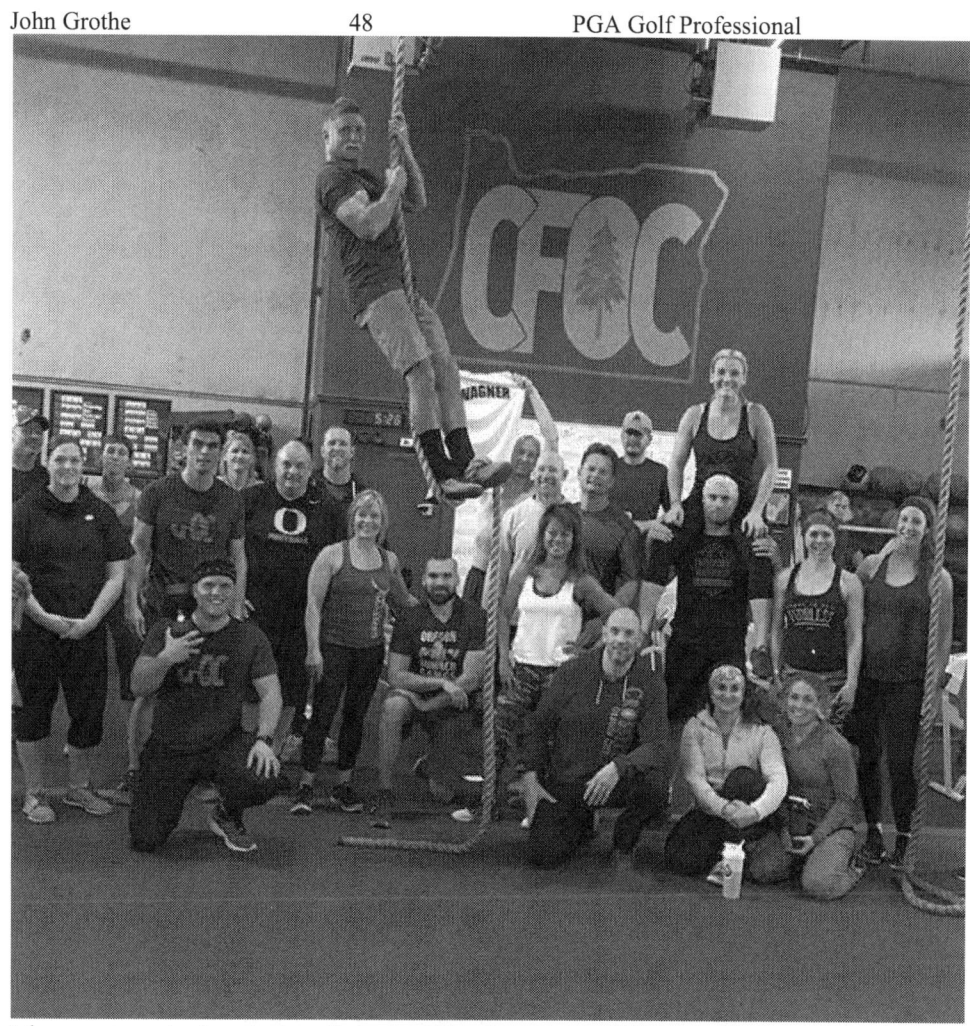

John Grothe   48   PGA Golf Professional

John grew up enjoying playing all sports. When he got out of HS he decided to compete in golf for his college. He was successful at it and went on to make it his career.

When he was 27 his father died. He became borderline depressed and he gained weight. He had a son, Colton, who was dealing with health issues and he became isolated and even heavier.

He saw the strength in Colton and decided to challenge himself. He found CFOC and his initial reaction was "What the heck? No desk. No mirrors. I guess I'll have to find my own way." He said that Scott was great. He realized that he was weak and out of shape. But Scott encouraged him and built the foundation of good movements and mechanics. He said he got his ass whipped every day – that he had a lot to learn – and he made the commitment to improve every day.

John stated that the community truly welcomed him – it is what keeps him coming back. Everybody is treated the same. Never say "I can't." Say, "I am working on this." Success came out of the community. He said that Jen would kick his ass if she saw him not giving his full effort.

He had a change in attitude, was making progress, and working out of his depression.

His son, Colton, has epilepsy. He has two or more seizures a day. He will always need a caretaker. It is socially isolating and difficult to be part of that dynamic. Colton had an attack that created almost continuous seizures. He was in the hospital and there seemed to be no way to address the attacks. The Children's Cancer Association (CCA) heard of Colton's condition and offered help in the form of music that seemed to sooth Colton.

John told Jen about what was happening, and Jen took it and ran with it. She created the "Colton WOD" as a way for the community to support CCA and Colton. She found community businesses who agreed to donate a certain dollar amount for every rep completed during a day-long workout at CFOC.

John explained it like this: Epilepsy is socially excluding and separating and exceedingly difficult for the child and the family. The CFOC family is exactly the opposite. It allows me to belong and to stay positive. Colton has become a rallying point for CFOC.

The Colton WOD is long, hard, and arduous. It symbolizes Colton's battle. It re-charges the family and has a direct effect on Colton. We all deal with something, John says. The response caused by CFOC was massive and overwhelming. CCA provides services for Colton and music to calm and support him.

CFOC does the Colton WOD annually and supports other efforts to raise funds for CCA.
John says the three most positive things in his life are Colton's courage, CFOC, and CCA.
And, he said with tears in his eyes, Jen called Colton an athlete.

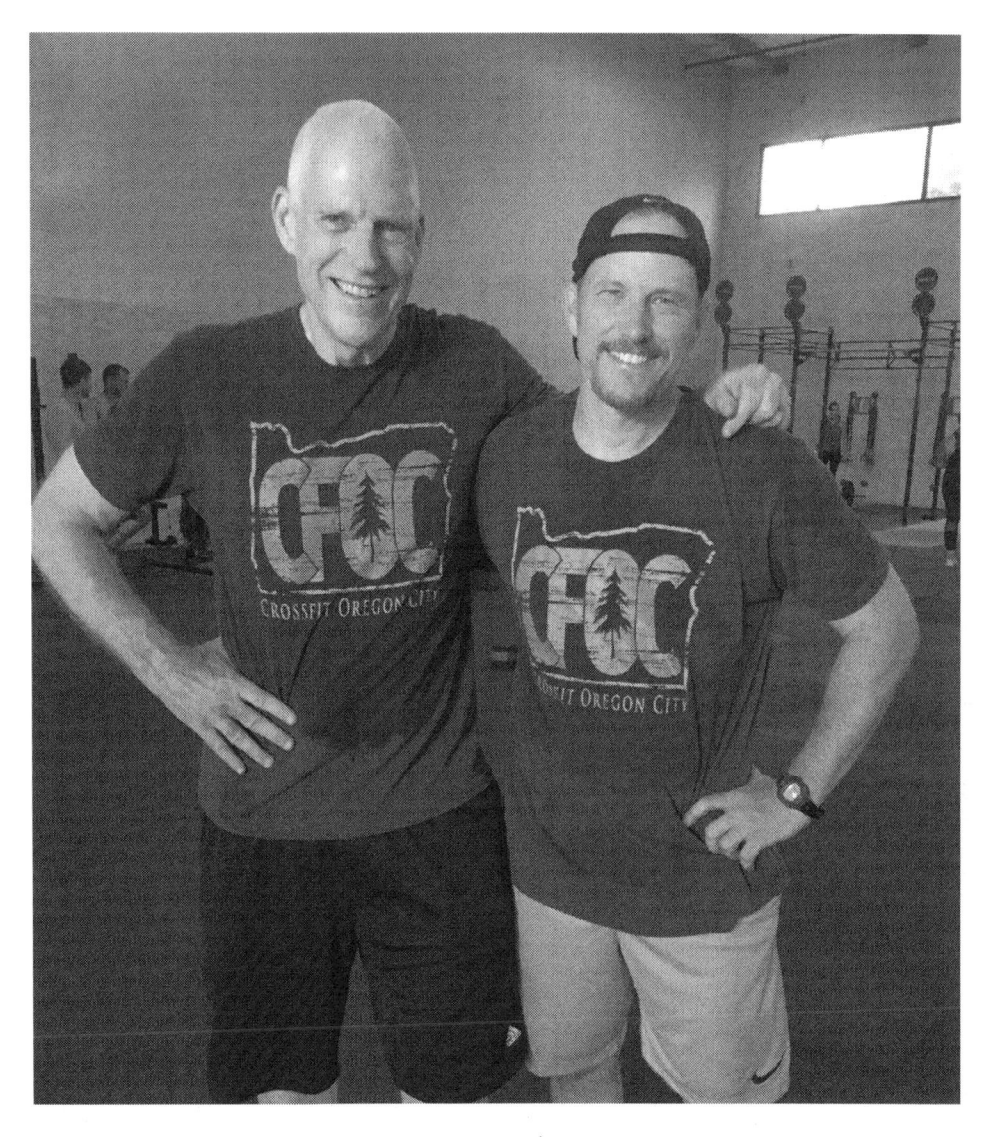

Today's workout is the second celebration of the 7th Anniversary of the start of CFOC. Mark is the coach for the workout, and he cannot get through the explanation of the elements of the workout without Jen correcting him. This seems to be their habit when Mark coaches 🙂

I am partnering with the other Todd A. Weber! I think this is the first time we have worked out together. The workout promises to be a doozey.

We start with 7 rounds of 7 cal row and 7 kettle bell swings. Todd is a fast rower and I am hitting a personal best speed. It goes amazingly fast. Then we run 200 m.

The next element is 7 rounds of 7 lateral burpees over the rower with 7 box steps. Then we run 200 m.

Then comes 7 rounds of alternate dumb bell snatches and 7 squats. Then we run 200 m. I am starting to feel this now.

Next is 7 rounds of 7 single overhead dumb bell presses with 7 plyo pushups. We run 200 m. Now it really has my attention.

Then we do 7 rounds of 7 hang cleans and 7 shoulder to overhead. We run 200 m. Except that it is more of a walk than a run as this round really took it out of me. Todd is looking good and going strong.

Then comes 7 rounds of 7 sit-ups and 7 wall balls. We run 200 m. For me this is a needed respite as I can do these movements well.

The last element is 7 rounds of 7 burpee box jumps and 7 burpee pullups. It is a killer and we get halfway through when time runs out. 40 minutes of sweat and trying to catch my breath.

Todd has been able to keep a good pace and do well throughout the workout. It has kicked my butt. I am so glad we got to work out together. He is truly a good person and I like him a lot.

Stacy Juratovac   52   massage therapist/cosmetology

Stacy is a cheerful, hardworking woman. She tends to keep to herself along with her long-time friend Teri. They both tend to sneak in quietly, do the workout and then disappear before you can say "hi." They are part of the 9 AM class and I have grown to know and love them.

Stacy was active when she was younger. She did cheer in high school and was a gym member for quite a while after that. She was introduced to Jen and decided to try CFOC in 2013. She said that she got her ass whipped at first and that she was very shy, so she tended to stay alone.

Her family encouraged her to stay and she decided to keep the commitment she had made to herself. She works out 5 days a week. She was diagnosed with breast cancer in 2015.

She continued to work out and "came to be normal." It was safe. The day of her surgery there was total support from CFOC and workouts done all over the crossfit community for "The EveryDay Warriors" who have cancer. Her doctors told her that her recovery was much better because she was fit.

She started running and members ran with her – she was smiling broadly when she said that. She said that it's a family. It is welcoming. There is so much support. It is a great place.

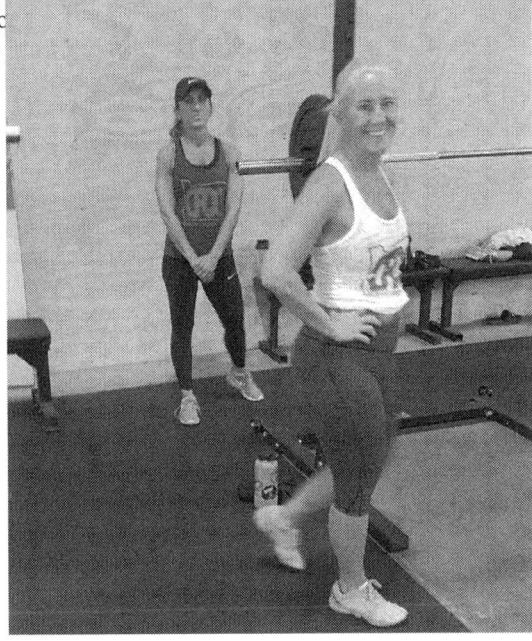

This is   gement. There is such a great connectic

James Wolfe-McCormack   36   Special Ed teacher CFOC coach

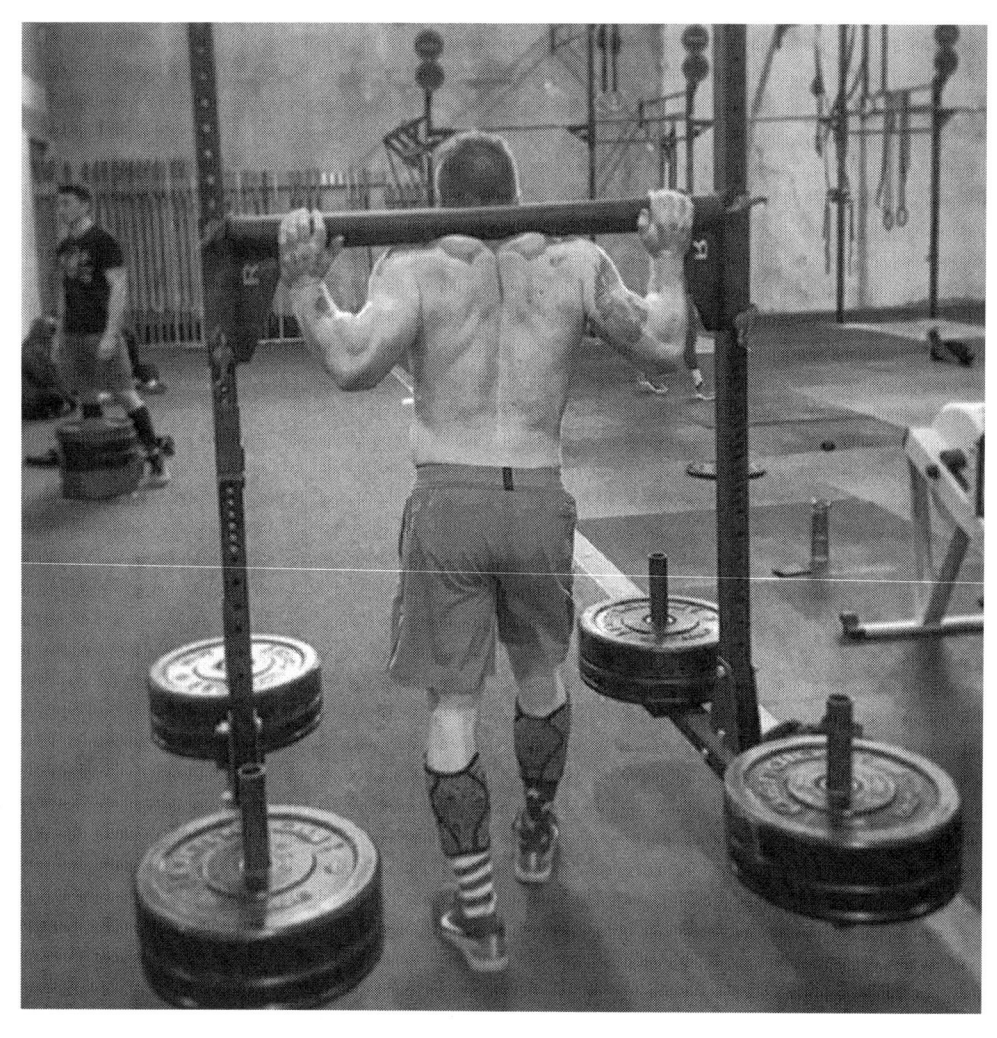

James is a special individual. He warms my heart every chance I get to talk with him.

James grew up a military brat. He moved a lot and played sports a lot. He was into soccer, baseball, HS football. He calls himself a utility man. As a senior in high school it was discovered he had cancer. Part of his self-care in beating cancer was to become active in fitness.

He started lifting weights at 24 Hr. Fitness. He became involved in roller derby. And he went to college to become a teacher. He found crossfit when his roller derby team was training for the national championships. He said that it was a great fit.

Then he discovered that he has Type I Diabetes. That was the end of his roller derby dreams.

His wife discovered CFOC 4 years ago and suggested that they get active again. He fell in love with crossfit. He says that it helped him to reflect on self and his family and where he is going with his life. He found it mentally and physically challenging. He says that CFOC is incredibly open and warm – it felt like a family.

James says you will get fit and you will meet good people. There is always something new to learn. He found a small group of special people that he calls his social therapy debrief. They work out early Saturday mornings together. He is always excited for Saturday mornings.

James says that Jen is like extended family. He has plans to reflect on how cross fit extends into other parts of his life. He is working on keeping fueled. He is looking to develop more endurance and strength. He leaves the box and is hungry for more.

And, he says that crossfit helps him manage his diabetes. He is off the pump and using shots. He has decreased his use of insulin.

He loves to share his story. He says it is a story of hope. He loves to coach and compete. He is a special guy. He is one of my Heroes.

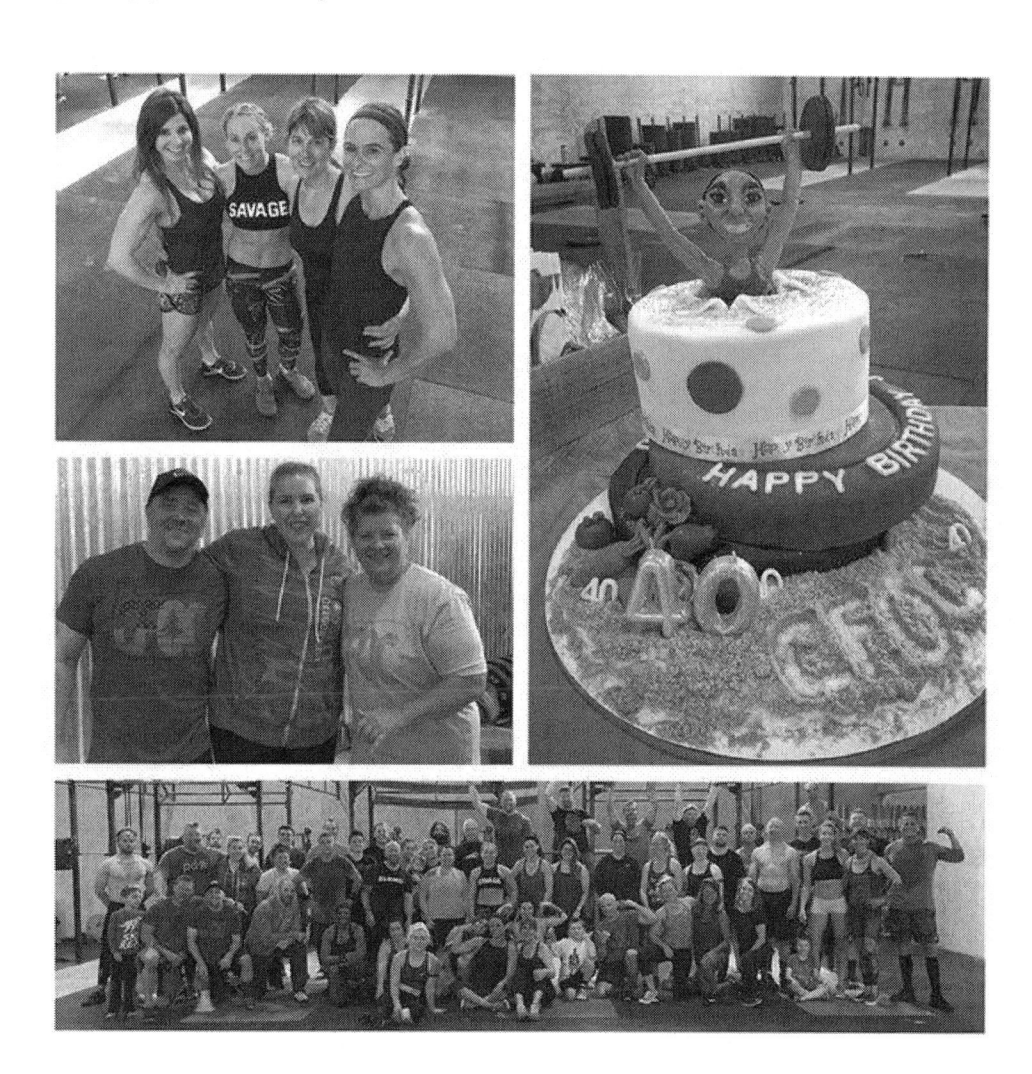

That is the purpose of these kinds of workouts… To celebrate and/or to remember and/or to support. And to have fun with good people.

There are other WODs during the year that support cancer and other causes. It is the nature of Jen and Scott to give what they can, and the box responds as well. It is a very moving dynamic and makes it so meaningful to be part of this community.

Chapter Twelve

Purpose

Victor Frankl, in the book *Man's Search for Meaning*, talks about a sense of purpose being a powerful force for health. Based on his experiences/observations in the Nazi concentration camps during the Second World War, Frankl postulated that purpose provides a means for rising above circumstances and conditions to be more capable to take helpful action.

His observations and conclusions were later confirmed by a wide-spread research project with survivors of POW camps during the Korean conflict. People with a sense of purpose have lower morbidity and mortality rates than those in similar or the same situations who don't.

Purpose is a component of health that is overlooked by many, but for us it must be considered as a connection to a more robust, meaningful aging process.

Frankl and others found that the sense of purpose does not need to be "big." It just needs to be meaningful. It can be about living out a spiritual or religious belief. Or it could be about providing for our family or community in some way. Or it could be about some small but important gesture that can help others.

It is certainly about finding something larger than ourselves that we can contribute to. As I mentioned earlier, it could be the aspirations we held earlier in life that were put aside with house payments, 2-car garages, putting kids through college, and trying to save for retirement.

Fitness and health may give us more capacity and tenacity to live more fully. What do we do with the expanded capacity? How are we to "spend" that renewed energy?

We know, or should know, that an extended and/or more robust aging process does not mean we do not have to face our own mortality. It gives us deeper questions to consider. And deeper commitment and focus to share.

Meditation on Death

The longer we are together
The larger death grows around us.

How many we know by now
Who are dead! We, who were young,
Now count the cost of having been…
Our hair turns white with our ripening
As though to fly away in some
Coming wind, bearing the seed
Of what we know. It was bitter to learn
That we come to death as we come
To love, bitter to face
The just and solving welcome
That death prepares. But that is bitter
Only to the ignorant, who pray
It will not happen. Having come
the bitter way to better prayer, we have
the sweetness of ripening.

Wendell Berry

    It is said that we come to wisdom too late in life for it to help. If we gain fitness and energy that allows time for us to contribute more, then our wisdom can be put to good use. And we have an obligation to share it.
    I think that along with more strength, balance, power, stamina, flexibility, mobility, and awareness of my body and how to use it well, I've gained a clearer understanding of how to apply my talents and capacities more effectively. This book is one aspect of that.
    What do you have to contribute? What have you to share that could make this world a little bit better each day? If you had the energy and capacity to give more, how would you use it?

Chapter Thirteen

The CFOC Tales

There are so many great stories about members of CFOC that I am going to arbitrarily categorize them and let them demonstrate the power and strength of this community.

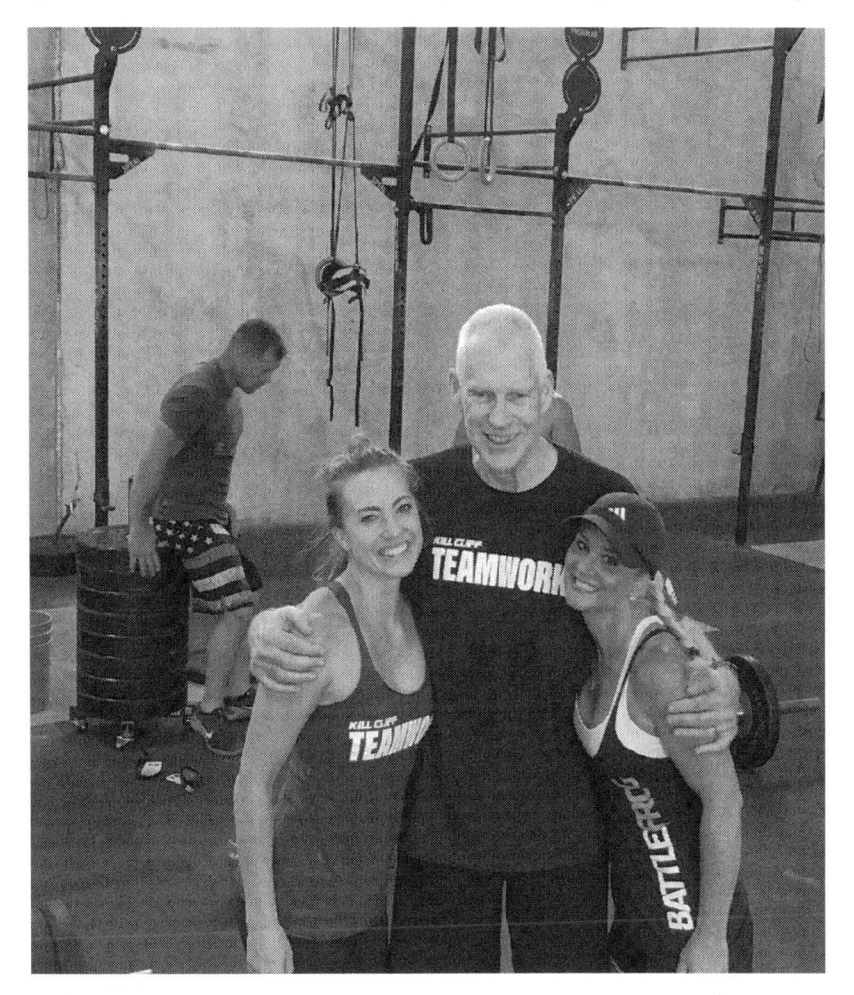

There are days that I wonder if I am always going to wake up stiff and sore from the previous day's workout. I keep thinking there will come a point when I am fit enough that I will move freely and gracefully without any reminders.

Then I realize that the stiffness and being sore is a sign of progress. It is a gift. It shows that my body is still learning and changing to adapt to the new conditions I'm demanding of it. It is a sign that even though I am 69 years old, my body can still grow new muscle and still create more flexibility and mobility. I can become better every day. It may not be as fast or easy as it once was, but if I keep working, keep lifting, keep stretching, keep moving a little past my comfort zones every day, I can improve. That is a great realization! It doesn't stop if I keep working. It makes me wonder how far I can take this.

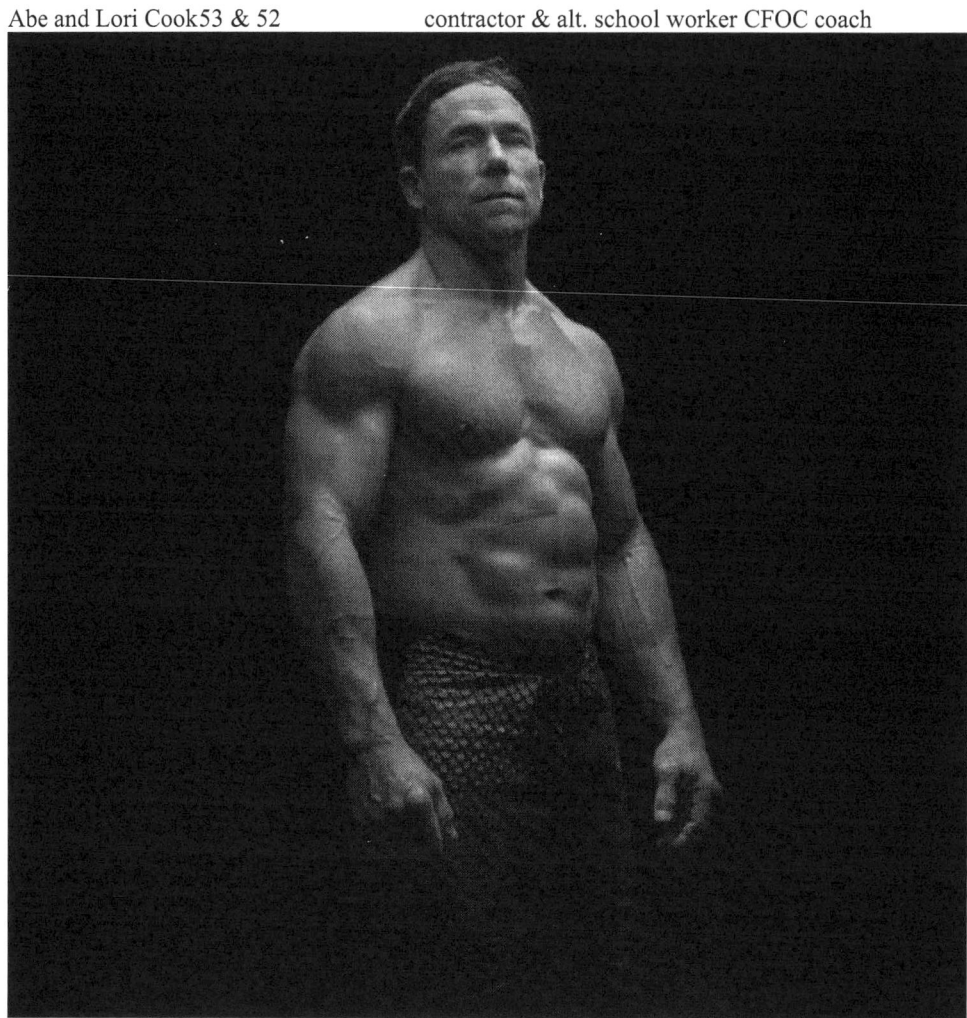

Abe and Lori Cook 53 & 52   contractor & alt. school worker CFOC coach

I was not sure what to expect when I interviewed Abe and Lori. If there is an alpha male at CFOC, Abe is probably the man. And Lori is an imposing athlete as well.

I met Abe a couple of times before the interview – just enough to say "hi." My expectations were that he and Lori were probably stand-offish and a bit arrogant, given their status in the box. It could not have been further from the truth.

Lori and Abe are so warm and engaging I felt like we were best friends in minutes. They are humble, funny, honest, and open.

Abe was into sports when he was younger – baseball and wrestling in high school…then being on the rodeo circuit later. Lori said she was addicted to exercise. She tried every fad, she wanted to look good. She says she probably had an eating disorder and after her son was born, she worked out all the time.

They found cross fit and Abe didn't like it at first. At the beginning, you had to do burpees if you were late, and the workouts were hard. After two months both were surprised that they weren't bored. They made friends, they would talk on the way home, they would work out together – it was like date night.

They got interested in competition, the couples they met became a tight-knit group and it was like family. Abe said that if he was going to compete, he was going to put everything into it. They went to Bend for the summer games and Abe took 3rd place. A bunch of people from the box went to support him – "These are our people." It is a great fit for us. We've been to a lot of cross fit boxes and the whole cross fit community is tight. But this place is special!

There is a high level of mutual respect and admiration. "My circle is where it needs to be." Both Lori and Abe say they have never stayed with something this long. It is the people – and it is our time to be together. They both like the aspect of continuing to improve, getting better, and looking good. It is the ultimate playground.

Abe has competed at the regional and crossfit games levels. A few years ago, he finished 8th in his age group at the CrossFit Games. Their whole family is fit and involved with crossfit. This year he finished 5th in the world for his age group in the Crossfit Open.

The picture of Abe you see here hangs in the office at CFOC where I conducted interviews. People would come in and say, "If you want to look like Abe, you have to eat like Abe." I asked Lori if that is true. She laughed saying, "No way!" He out works what he eats. Seeing Abe do a workout, I am not sure there are many people who can work that hard.

Today's workout seems like a nice change of pace. It is a repeat of a workout we've done twice this year. It is a good measure of where we are.

It starts with tempo squats – 5 count down, 3 hold, then up for 5 reps – 4 times. I am using a 20# kettle bell and it is making my legs shake.

Then we do Helen (some crossfit workouts are named - the ones with women's names tend to be very tough). For me that is three rounds of 200m run, 21 kettle bell swings (35#) and 12 pull ups. I do it in 9:47, which is much quicker than last time. Things are looking up.

Matt Stewart

Matt is a pleasant young man who started at CFOC about 1 and 1/2 years ago. He had been a member previously, but his wife at the time was not happy with his time at the box. It became complicated and he stopped coming.

He is back now after a divorce and is happy to be here. He said the first week back was brutal, the challenge and the people and the community "makes me happy." It is positive, It is infectious – all being on the same journey. It is a lot more than fitness. It feels like a party.

He said that it is close-knit – a true community. He has met someone he is dating. He is socializing, playing pool, going to BBQs. He said that he went to a regular gym and never met anyone.

He said that for him it is the lifestyle that is so attractive. It is positive, healthy, and people live according to their values. He says he even likes working out with the "old guys" like me.

In the short time Matt has been back, he has become so buff it is crazy. He has become one of my favorite people.

Today's workout is a continuation of the benchmark WODs. Matt plays a featured role in this workout ⍰ After a class warm-up with barbells, we do a barbell combination for 5 rounds. The combination is 3 dead lifts, 2 cleans, and 1 shoulder to overhead. Being a combination means we do it all without putting the bar down. Brad is the coach and he is on a mission to insure everyone is using good form.

He spots Matt using a strict press to get his weight overhead. He asks Matt why. He should be using a slight dip and powering the bar up with his legs. Matt shakes his head and says that is the way he has always done it. That is not what you want to say to Brad.

Matt and Brad spend about 5 minutes working on helping Matt get his legs into the lift. One of Brad's favorite sayings is, "You don't lift with your arms, you lift with your legs!"

We finish the lifting set after 5 rounds and after Matt almost hurt himself by getting the bar up so high that he almost lost control. He laughs but you can tell it was not what he expected.

Then we do "Grace." This is a workout of 30 clean and jerks for time. It is one of the workouts that critics of crossfit like to point to as being dangerous. Critics claim that doing Olympic lifts for speed is an invitation to bad form and injury. They do not consider a couple of important factors. One is that the weight is set for males and females at a relatively low amount. Even that amount may be too high for Brad if he feels you cannot do the 30 reps safely.

The second factor is having a coach like Brad. He drills good form into us over and over...like today doing form work right before the WOD. And he drills into us to use lower weights when we are lifting for repetitions.

We are split into two groups: one to count reps while the other lifts and then the reverse. My form is not good enough to do high repetitions for time, so I will be doing one arm alternative dumb bell snatches for time. It is much safer, and I will be using a relatively low weight.

I count for Tyler the first round. He worked out at his job last night (He works for 24 HR Fitness) but wants to see if he can push it for a new best time. He starts out strong, but at 13 or 14 reps he starts to lose form and to struggle. I remind him about what Brad said – use your legs to lift. He guts out another 10 reps. People come over to encourage him and he puts together another 5 reps to finish at 4:40. He is totally spent when he is done.

I am thinking that maybe I picked too much weight for my turn. We get set up to start the next round. Tyler will count for me. I have a 30# dumb bell. We start. I have a nice pace going and feel strong. I am concentrating on keeping my core tight, back straight and the dumb bell close to my body. At around 24 reps, I can't seem to get my breath. I don't quite panic, but it is a very strange feeling trying to get oxygen into my lungs and not being able to do it. I finish the 30 reps in 1:37.

When I recover enough to talk, I say to Tyler that I should have used a heavier weight. He smiles and says given that I couldn't breathe the last few reps, it was probably the perfect amount for this time. Jen said later that I needed to use more weight ☒

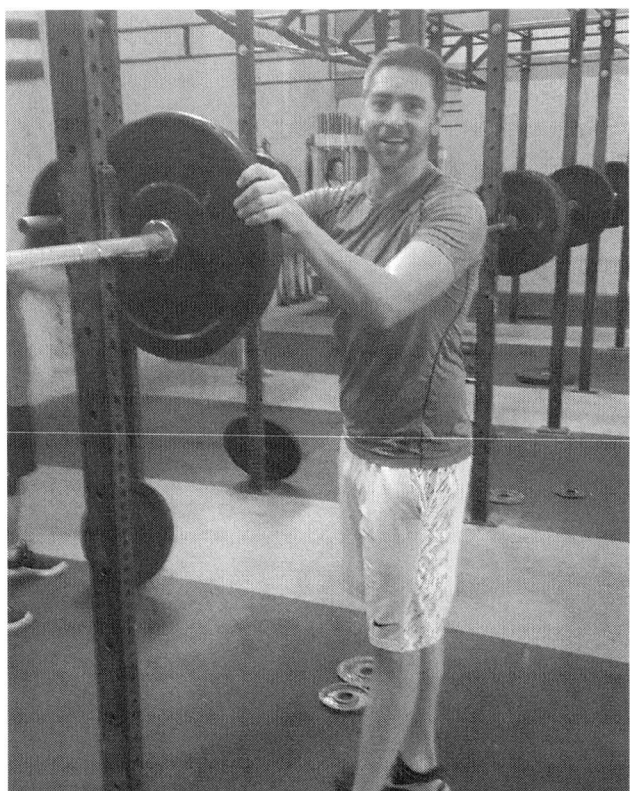

The next morning, we are faced with a "Four Girls" WOD – Diane, Karen, Annie, and with the time left AMRAP of Cindy. We are celebrating girls' week. All the benchmark workouts are named after women. There is something perverse in that.

It is a partner workout and I have Sue as a partner. It will be fun. We start with splitting 21 – 15 – 9 reps of deadlifts and handstand push-ups. Since neither one of us can do HSPUs, we substitute dumb bell presses. It goes well – feeling fairly good.

Then comes "Karen," which is infamous in crossfit circles. It is 150 wall balls. I have not done Karen before and even with a partner it gets tough.

Then we are on to Annie – 50, 40, 30, 20, 10 reps of jump rope double-unders and sit ups. Again, we can't do double-unders, so I do jumping jacks and Sue does singles, and we both do the sit ups. The number of reps makes this one more of a challenge. We finish with lots of time left on the 30-minute clock to do Cindy.

Cindy is 5 pull ups, 10 pushups (hand release so the chest touches the floor) and 15 air squats. We start by alternating full rounds but by the third or fourth round we are both struggling with the 10 pushups. So for that, every round we split the pushups. The air squats are tough after the wall balls. It is a good, tough struggle to finish.

Sue and I are happy with our work. We pushed it hard. It was fun. There was no taking it easy on this one!

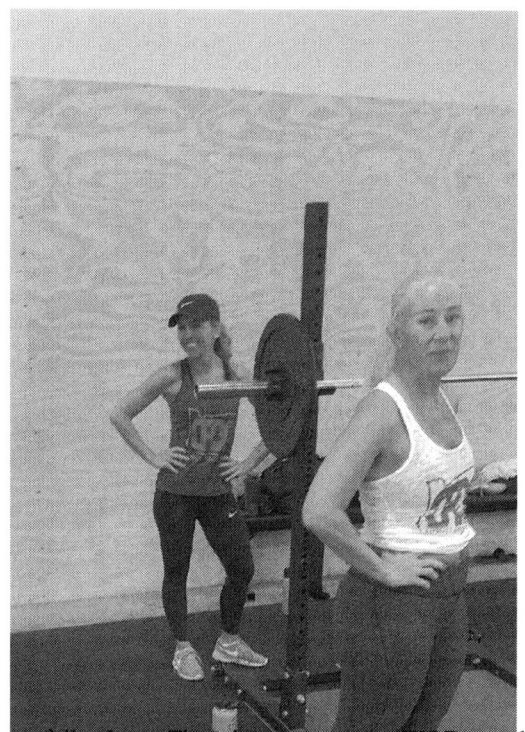

Teri and Stacy are awfully close. They do every partner WOD together if they are both here. Stacy talked with Teri about coming to CFOC for a long time, but she didn't feel she could do it until her last girl finished high school.

Teri was active when she was younger. She has always been active in cheer, dance and the performing arts. She started weightlifting as a dancer to gain upper body strength and to have balance. She thinks her lack of injuries as a dancer is due to her weight work.

She wants to make the most of what she was given, and she wants to support her friend, Stacy, as much as she can. She says she has found a whole new set of friends – a "good crew of chicks."

She says that she does not ask a lot from her family and this is something she really wanted to do. I need to go. I want to shape up!

She says that she died when she started. She was intimidated, wanted to hide in the back. She jokes that it was hard to face that as a professional performer she danced in front of thousands but when it came to crossfit she wanted to hide.

She says that after a year, she is feeling like she "got it." She wants to take it up a notch. She says this helps with every aspect of her life and that it is wonderful that Scott and Jen "want us to find our best."

She is making new friends. Everybody cheers each other on! It is so positive and accepting. You can "find your brave." The love is so strong. It is an even playing field for women – it is a life saver.

I've gotten to know Teri a bit over the past year and enjoy her warmth and sense of humor. It is a joy to watch the love and friendship shared between Teri and Stacy.

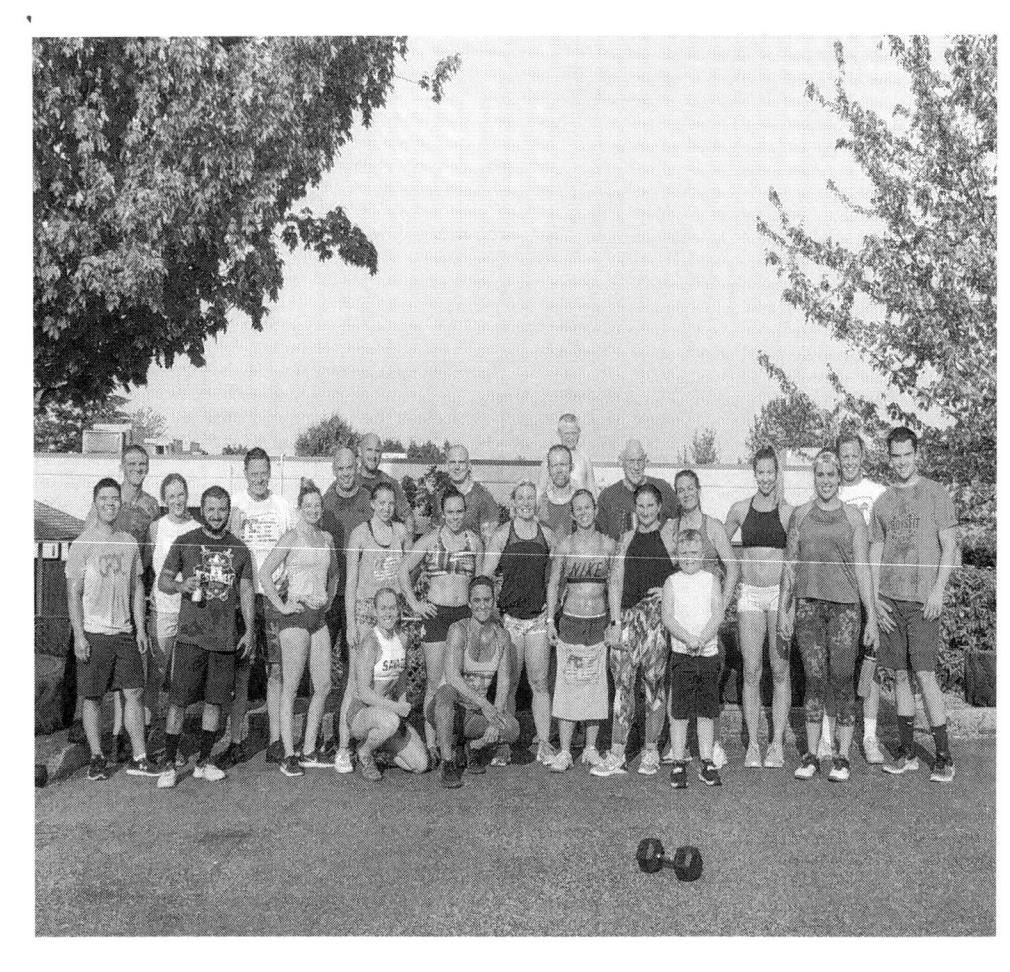

Aside –

There is an aspect of the crossfit community that is about what drives us as adults to seek meaning, fulfillment, mastery, and autonomy. Daniel Pink, in his book "Drive" talks about the motivations that we all share. Once our basic needs are met, we look for ways to fulfill our higher aspirations.

Sometimes we can find a way to do this through work. Yet there are very few workplaces that give us an opportunity to self-direct the ways we can express these drives.

Crossfit is a place that allows us the opportunity to pursue these drives and gives us a meaningful container through fitness – and the community.

We can gain mastery through fitness. Learning and mastering movements, lifts, stamina, agility, and more. There is no end to the process as even after mastery there is more to learn, more to practice, more to become. It provides the "ultimate playground" as Abe Cook said. It is fun. It is challenging. It is useful and functional.

Autonomy is built both through gaining fitness and applying it. We decide what we want to focus on. It is not just the physical aspect of crossfit that gives us independent choices. It is the mental, emotional, and spiritual aspects as well.

Autonomy is also built by making the decisions about joining the community and about what kind of member one wants to be. Most of the time, we join groups automatically – bringing the person we are most comfortable with as our persona. However, in safe environments, where there is acceptance, support, and warmth we can be our "real selves" and join the community at a much deeper level.

In crossfit, we are all vulnerable. We are all pushing the limits of our comfort zones. We are all testing ourselves in ways that we have not since we were kids. We are open to experiencing the world through new senses that are bright and alive and vivid. This gives us the opportunity to build relationships in a different way.

And lastly there is meaning or purpose. By being engaged in a community of shared values, we can join in contributing in a way that is larger than ourselves. We can make a difference. We can make our lives count in a truly meaningful way.

As we discussed earlier, Victor Frankl, in "Man's Search for Meaning," talks about how having a purpose – seeking meaning – can be the most powerful form of motivation there is. It does not have to be deadly serious. It just needs to captivate our imagination and spirit enough to help shape our goals.

Crossfit is a natural goal machine. We want to change something. We want to improve something. We want to re-shape something. And all the people around us want that too! There is no dogma about how we set our goals. There is no prescribed way to be. There is no absolute belief system we must adopt.

We choose to be with people we like and who are doing things we like to do and who want to contribute to making things a bit better than they are currently. That is magic!

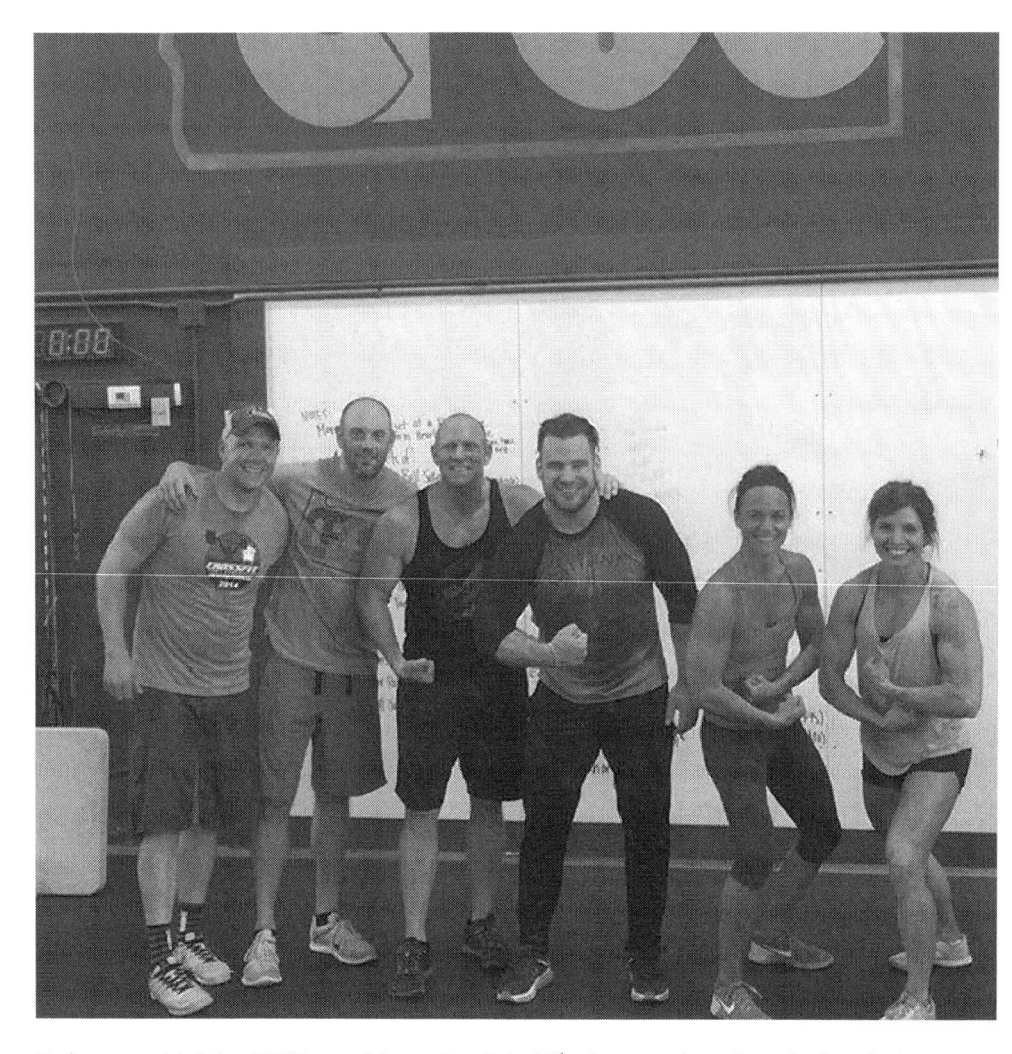

Today was a birthday WOD to celebrate Janelle's 30th. Jen must have been feeling devious because this workout was a killer. I got to partner with Matt for the first time in a while. He is so strong it is a mental challenge for me to picture being a good partner for him, but I am determined to do my best (I also had a little extra motivation based on a discussion some members of CFOC were having online – more about that later).

It is a thirty-minute partner workout with the reps split any way the partners choose. I have a good warm up because I was a half an hour early. We get set up. Then it is 3-2-1 go!

The first element is 30 squat cleans. Matt is going heavy and I'm still working on form – but it is still intense. We split it 5-5-5-5-5-5.

Then it is 8 rounds of 18 deadlifts, 19 burpee box jumps, and 88 double-unders. I am working on keeping my back flat for the deadlifts, so it is a good workout for me. I do 75#s and Matt does some huge weight. The burpee box jumps are more of an issue. I was able to jump to a 12-

inch box a couple of weeks ago but this time I am stumbling so I do step-ups. Matt is jumping to a 24-inch box. Then Matt does double-unders and I do jumping jacks.

We split the rounds 5-5-4-4 reps for deadlifts, 5-5-5-4 reps for burpee box jumps, and 44-44 for the double-unders. We start off with a really good pace. In the middle of the second round, Matt's jump rope falls apart, so I do extra jumping jacks while he finds a new rope.

We do not lose much time and are right back in rhythm for the 3rd round. Then Matt has trouble with the new rope because it is too short. He says the heck with it and does singles.

During the next round, Scott comes over to tell me to not soften my back on the last rep of the deadlifts when I put the bar down. I had not noticed that I was doing that. You learn something new every time. It is amazing.

Rounds 5 and 6 were getting tough. The burpee box jumps were taking their toll and I was feeling it. Matt seemed to be going well. Scott called out 1 minute and then the last 3 seconds and we were done. We completed 7 rounds and 10 reps. I was disappointed because I wanted to finish all 8 rounds. Matt was good with it. He is such an easy-going guy and I really enjoy working out with him. We talked for a few minutes about his dad, as I thought he might want to come to the box. I learned that his dad is disabled, and Matt has been taking care of him for quite a while. I told him whenever it made sense I would love to visit.

Matt says that he loves working out with me because I motivate him. I don't know what to say to that. I am just in awe of the good people who are part of CFOC, and I love being around Matt.

Lifting class is next. It has been a while since I've been to one. I am not sure why – probably because there have not been many lately. Brad and Scott are coaching.

Most of the people in the class are competitors going to the Best in the West competition at the end of the week. They will be building up to max lifts as their last hard training before going. I will be concentrating on form for the clean.

Once again it is about my back, chest and shoulders being in the right positions. Brad and Scott help until they get caught up with the competitors and Sara works with me to help feel the right way to set up. I have made a lot of progress, but it is still frustrating when I can't just do it right ⏤ I know it is a process. I know I need to be consistent in working on it. And I want to be able to do it now!

Sara helps a lot and I get into my set position much better. I have a few good lifts and Scott says he is happy. If he is happy, I am happy. So, I pack up and say goodbye.

I have such a calm feeling of joy and satisfaction as I leave. It was a good workout that kicked my butt and I got to know Matt a little better. I learned a couple of new things today. I made progress on my lifts. It is really good stuff.

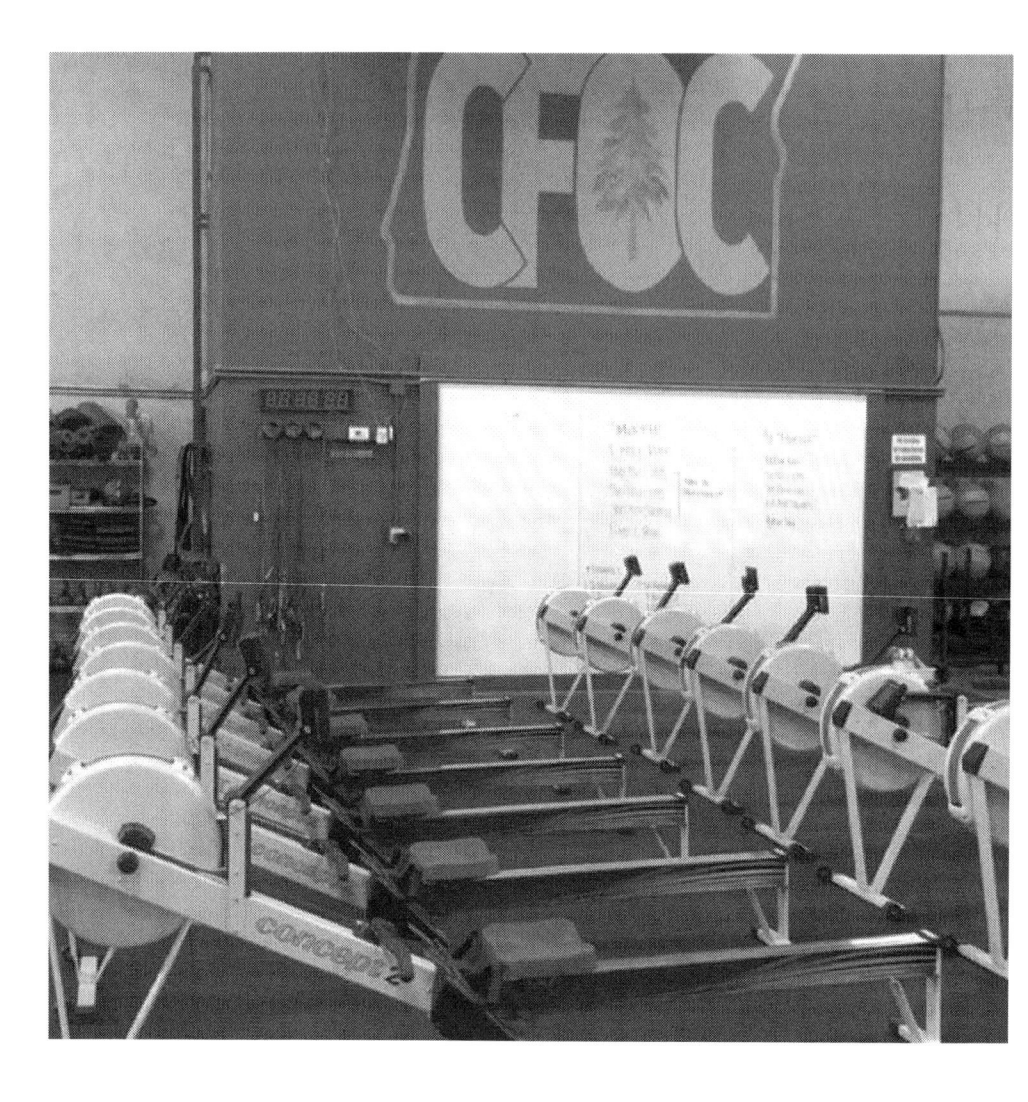

As I mentioned earlier, there is an interesting discussion going on in Facebook. One of the members wrote about seeing other members post workout results that did not accurately reflect what they did. It was a well-written plea for accuracy and honesty because the results are used for a number of reasons – WOD programming, setting times and weights, comparing results with others in other classes – and is used to measure one's progress over time. If the posted results are inaccurate, it can impact all those things. And it can create unrealistic expectations for inexperienced members.

There was an immediate response of varied intensity. Some wanted names of the offenders. Some thought it wasn't that important. Some thought it was a reflection on the whole community and wanted a more ethical stance.

I took it as an opportunity to examine my own approach to workouts and decided that I had been slacking in a few areas. There are movements that I could do as described but continued to do as scaled because it was easier and faster. I told myself that the intensity was still equal because I was doing them faster than what I could the true movement. However, I think that was just rationalization to avoid the harder movement.

So, I resolved to start doing the described movements whenever possible. It is the only way I will get better at those movements and that I will be able to get the designed benefits of the workout.

I started with burpees – which I had been doing to a box – and immediately realized how much more difficult it is than what I had been doing. I will start working on double-unders. I told myself they are not important because when am I going to go jump-roping down the street to save an infant? But, they are a benchmark movement for a reason, and I have been avoiding learning to do them. Time to start.

I don't think this was an intended result of the member's post, but it was good practice for me to review my approach and make changes where it made sense.

This may be one of those shadow areas that I was referring to earlier. I don't think it has a big impact on the community. But it did generate quite a bit of energy.

Today was one heck of a day. We did a birthday WOD for Kelii who is 45. It was hard.

Tiny partnered with me again. He is so strong, and I do not want to be a handicap for him as a partner, so I tend to push it as hard as I can when we workout together. The workout went like this:

45 cal row shared
45 overhead power snatches (extremely hard even with a light weight because of lack of shoulder mobility)
At 5 minutes 45 cal row
45 overhead squats – hard for the same reason
At 10 minutes 45 cal row
45 synchronized burpee box step overs
At 15 minutes 45 cal row (this one, I had to break early as I ran out of gas)
45 alternate dumb bell snatches
At 20 minutes 45 cal row

It actually didn't go this smoothly because we had to finish each set of 45 reps even if it was broken up by the row – which most movements were. Because of that, at 25 minutes we were still working on dumb bell snatches.

25 min 45 cal row
24 box step-overs
30 min stop

I was ruined when we stopped. It was so hard and so much fun at the same time. It was outrageous.

Then, I tripped over a weight and landed edgewise on a weight plate with my thigh. Man did that hurt! I am sure that there will be quite a bruise tomorrow. It drove home a point for me, though. I have enough muscle mass and bone density that I do not need to be overly concerned about falling. I am bruised. And I picked myself up and went to play golf with Tiny and his son. Not bad at 69.

Nutrition – Again

Eat meat and vegetables, nuts and seeds, some fruit, little starch, and no sugar. Keep intake at levels that will support exercise but not body fat.

Practice and train major lifts: deadlift, clean, squat, presses, clean and jerk, and snatch. Similarly, master the basics of gymnastics: pull-ups, dips, rope climbs, presses to handstands, pirouettes, flips, splits and holds. Bike, run, swim, row, etc. hard and fast.

Five or six days per week mix these elements in as many combinations and patterns as creativity will allow. Routine is the enemy. Keep workouts short and intense.

Regularly learn and play new sports.

Greg Glassman

It is important to note that as an older athlete I do not do most of the gymnastics movements. I either can't or don't want to chance an injury. My coaches find alternative movements, so I still get the intensity and benefit of the movements.

Do not think you can outwork a bad nutritional approach. It is harder and harder as we age to get past the effects of bad habits. Eating clean will set you up for success!

Chapter Fourteen

The Mitch Wagner Factor

Mitch is no longer a member of CFOC, but his presence is still felt every day. Mitch is a tremendous crossfit athlete who has qualified for the regionals for many years and who has come *this* close to going to the crossfit games. He has three regional banners flying in the box and many stories are told of his exploits.

During the Eastern regionals this year, all eyes were on the screen when Mitch was competing. Again, he came remarkably close to qualifying for the games.

He came to the box this week as he is visiting his parents, Don and Janine, who are members of CFOC. I had the chance to meet him and to watch him workout. I get it now! There is a big difference between the regular crossfit members and a regional and games athlete. He makes it look so easy and he is so strong and fast – it is amazing.

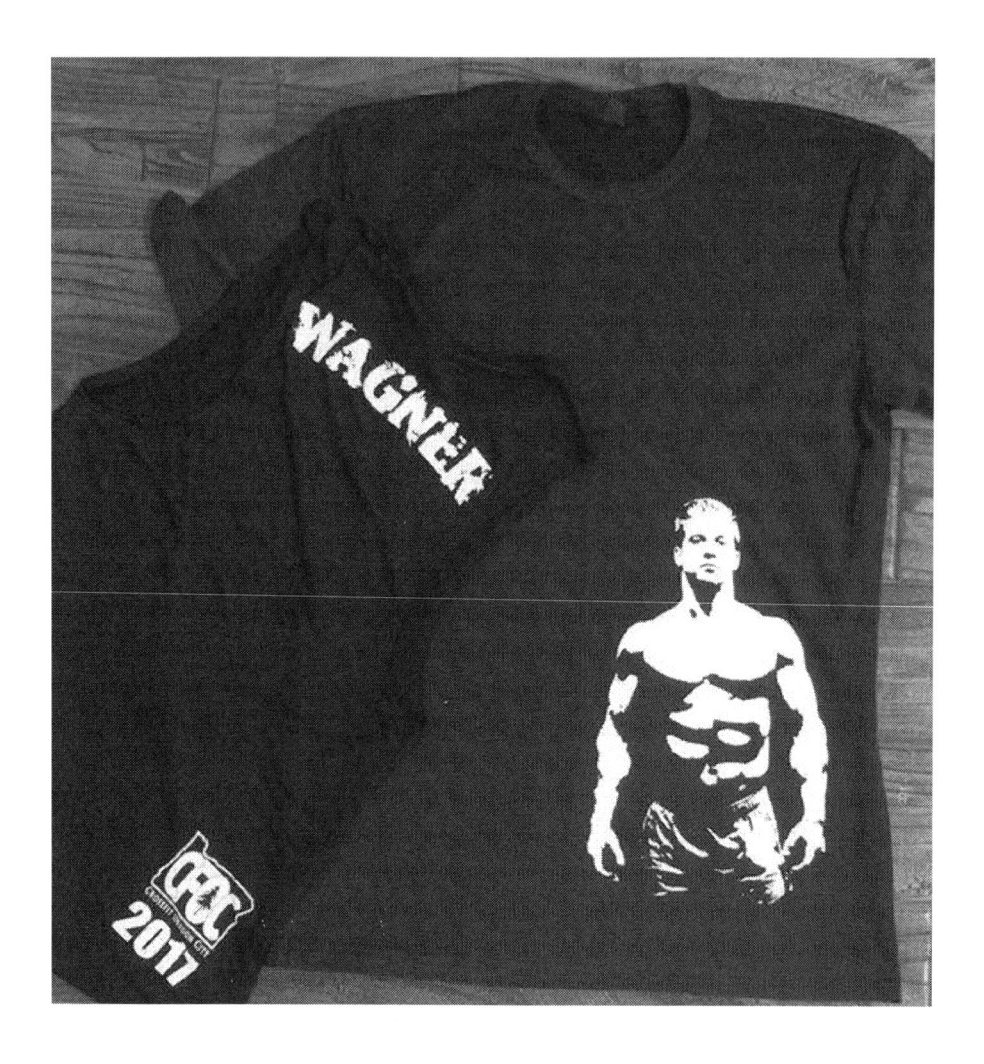

Janine Wagner   59   dental hygienist

Janine is a happy, beautiful soul. She is strong and determined and universally positive. She and Don, her husband, worked out together at the local Nautilus Gym and Janine was also active in walking and taking fitness classes. Don was still an active firefighter and he needed to be fit for his job.

They know Abe and Lori Cook who along with their son, Mitch, encouraged them to try crossfit. Mitch said to try it for a month – it will get easier.

Janine said that she was totally intimidated when she started. She has been coming to CFOC for 4 years now and wishes she started 25 years earlier.

She says that she likes how she feels. It helps with her anxiety. She was comfortable with the Cooks and it spread from there. It is family. It is hard to do, but there is so much support. Her journey has become to help others. She loves these people.

Janine was working out close to me when we were doing "Fran." That is the benchmark WOD of 21-15-9 thrusters and pull ups. Mitch has a video that is used to show how it can be done.

Janine was down to her last 4 pull ups. She was struggling a bit and finding it hard to get her chin over the bar because of fatigue. She would come close – but not quite make it. She did not give up! She kept pushing herself to finish the workout. After two or three tries for each rep, she was able to complete the WOD.

It was one of the most amazing things I've seen at the box. It would have been far easier to say, "that was close enough" and count the reps that did not quite make it over the bar. She did not. She didn't quit, and she didn't take a short cut. She finished. I was so impressed with her integrity and grit.

Both Don and Janine talked about what they planned to do when they are both retired (Don retired this past year). There were planning on moving South to the sun or moving closer to their family – Mitch in Georgia. Now, they said, they are planning on staying here where their friends and box are. It is family.

Today's WOD was a repeat from about 2 months ago. We are checking on progress and growth. It starts with deadlifts – 3 sets of 5 reps. I am still working on form but will go a little heavier. It feels good and I can push the weight up a bit.

The next part is 3 minutes on and 3 minutes off of 30 cal row and max burpees to a box – 5 rounds. During the 3 minutes on it is supposed to be a full sprint. I am doing the step ups to a 20" box for the first time and I forget to do the push-up part of the burpees for the first three rounds. I still push it as hard as I can, and finish drenched in sweat. Astin is there to talk to after the workout so it is a great day.

Don Wagner   59   retired fire fighter

Don is known for his huge biceps and his great mustache ☐ He was active as a kid working on the farm and played football through junior high school. He worked out at a gym and did some weight training, but found he was putting on weight. He had an experience in a fire rescue that convinced him he needed to do something to be more fit.

He had a buddy who did cross fit and Mitch, his son, found Jen and Scott, so he decided to try it with Janine. He went to a Saturday class and was the last guy finishing a workout. He was dying and yet, he said, people were so supporting. He liked it and he liked that it was so tough. He said that the coaches were great in helping him learn Olympic lifting, kettle bell work, and body weight work. It was so varied and so hard. No time to get bored. He said that he learned that form was so important, and it was refreshing to have coaches work with people individually.

His brother and sister passed from cancer and Jen made a special WOD for them. She also made a WOD celebrating Don's retirement. He says there is no judgment at the box. Everybody is encouraging and supportive. People really care!

He says that it is the fountain of youth. Don and Janine are both amazingly fit. When I grow up I want to have biceps as big as Don's.

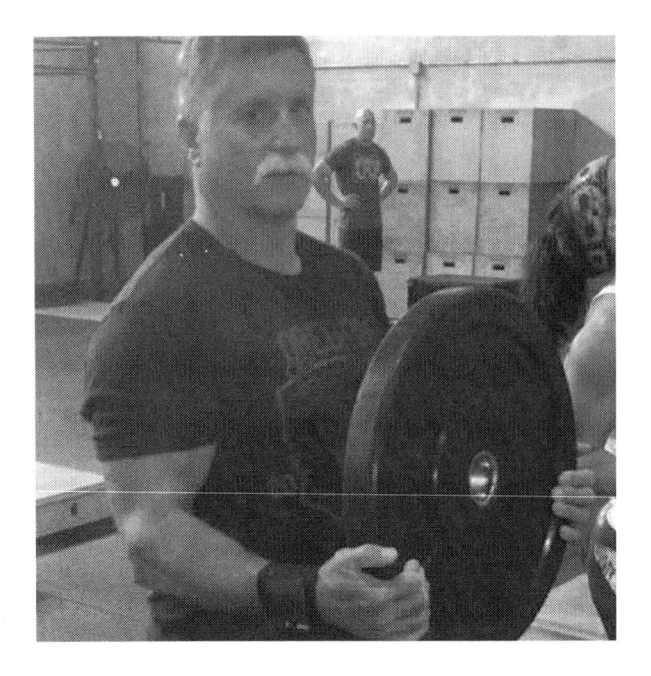

I am in Bend for the Best of the West competition. CFOC has competitors in almost every heat. It is exciting and confusing to watch. I think CFOC has the largest group of people here and certainly the most organized and vocal.

The workouts are hard – some even brutal. It is hard to keep track of where the different athletes are in the workouts.

I like to yell and support my friends, but I find myself wanting to compete. (I am competing this year). Not that I could yet. The movements and weights are way beyond my ability now. But I think I can do it if I keep progressing.

There are some excellent athletes here. And the crowd is a mixed bag. It is still a bit shocking to me to see friends and relatives of the athletes who do not take care of themselves. Here are people who are working their butts off to become as fit as possible and next to them are people who obviously are not ready yet.

I guess that is the way it is in any sport or activity. There are those who do it and there are those who watch. I want to do it. I want to push myself in a way that only competition can bring out. Not that I have any chance of "winning." It is not about that. It is about continuing to stretch my comfort zone and to push beyond what seems possible.

I saw Abe and Lori there cheering for their son-in-law Shane. He is a beast. Lori and I talked a bit about the conundrum of finding people who have the same interests as you but are not walking the same path. It can be comforting and supporting. And it can be isolating and lonely.

For me, I think some of it is that I have not been in a relationship for a while and I want to share these experiences with someone I care about. I am sure that I will find a nice crossfit lady to hang out with. Then this won't be an issue.

That is part of being in a community as well. It can be lonely being around people when you are "alone" in your personal life. I find myself being careful not to impose or seem needy. I feel like the odd man out at times. Yet, these are the closest people in my life. It is a question we all grapple with – how close is too close? Or is it only the introverts that have this struggle?

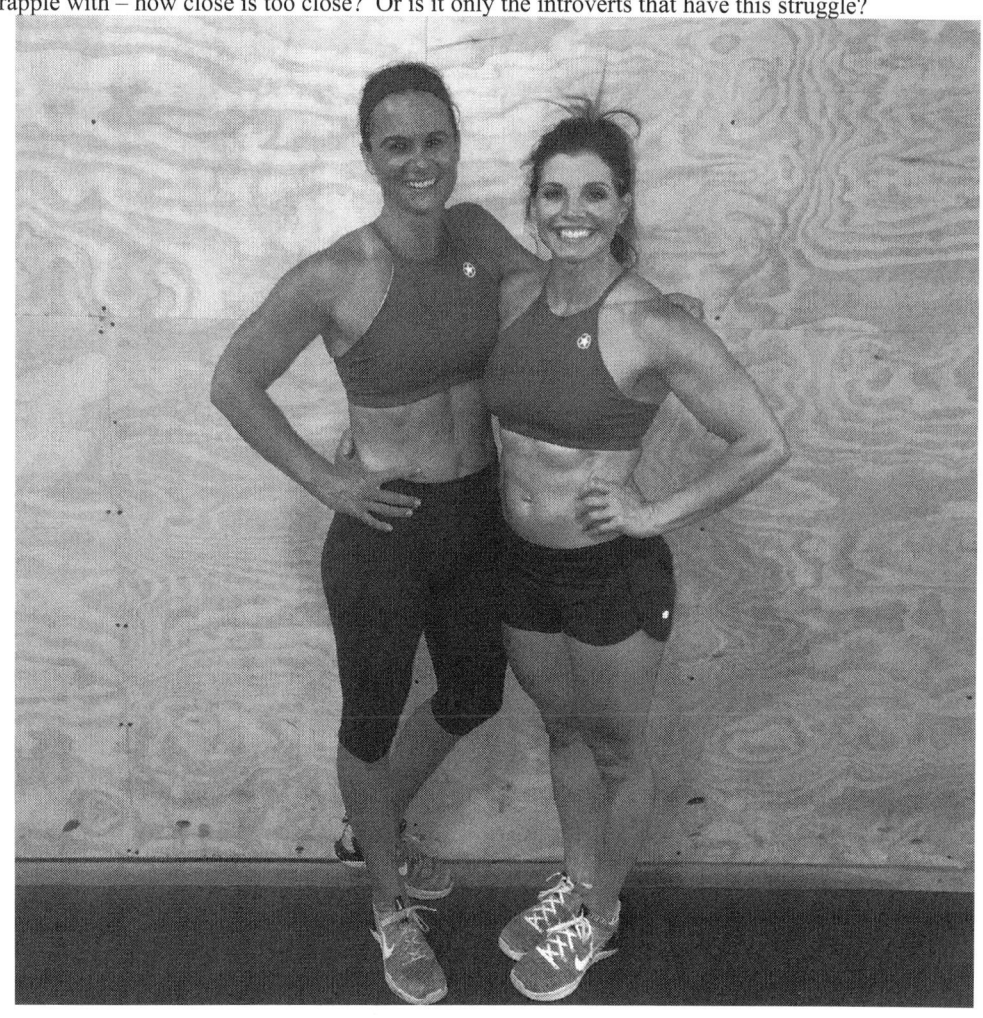

Dave Hjorten   69   retired diesel mechanic

Dave is back! He had a rough year. Cancer surgery and then hernia surgery laid him low for probably three months combined. He is back now and is as irascible as ever.

Dave was a high school football player and then went into the Navy during the Viet Nam conflict where he found weightlifting and swimming as fitness activities. He did heavy work in the Navy as a mechanic and followed that trade when he left the service.

He worked out at the local Nautilus Center, as many other CFOC members did, and finally quit in disgust when he got tired of how dirty the place was and with the lack of good teaching for the people who were hogging the weights.

His wife joined CFOC a couple of years earlier and he thought he would give it a try. He says it has been fun since the day he started. He talks about having a 40 yr old's mindset in an older body and how that caused him to push too hard a few times and made for a few setbacks. I can totally relate with him on that one 🙂

Dave talks about how the people are so good he would recommend it to anyone. Everyone cheers for each other and it is so supportive. He believes in the special WODs for cancer and the Heroes. His bout with cancer was made less damaging because he is fit. His surgeon told him, "You are in good shape. Stay that way!"

He says he just does what his wife tells him to do… like I am supposed to believe that. They come to the box at different times because she is still working. He says that Susan is the one who pushes him to show up.

Dave says that CFOC is special. He really enjoys the people. It is clean. Class time is great. It is a good community.

Dave is the oldest member of the box (I am second) and he is tough as nails. He is strong, lean, and moves very well. Most young men would be lucky to have his physique. And I can call him a friend.

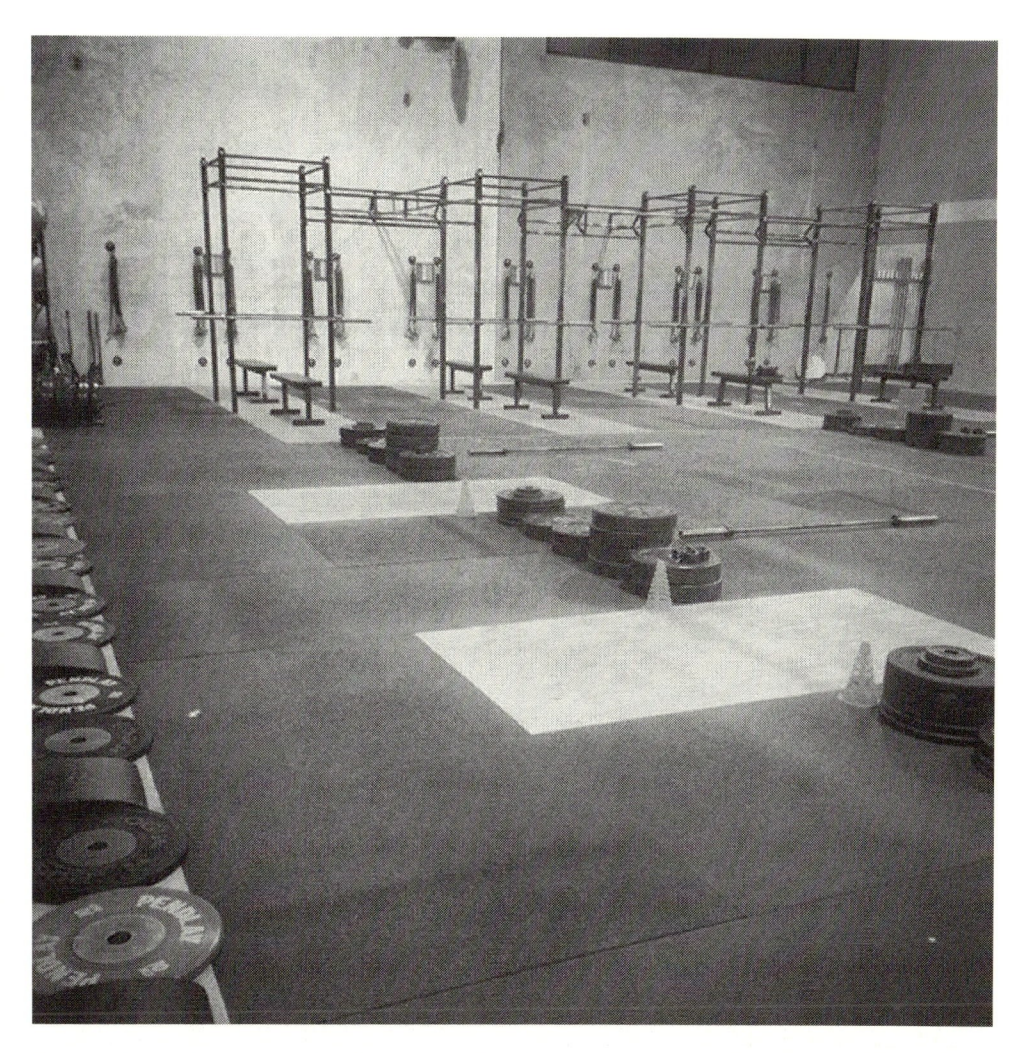

The workout today was tougher than usual. I think it was me and not the workout. Many of the folks who did the competition last weekend were back and it was fun to talk with them. I talked with Kelly about her experience with Emily doing the RX competition together. They looked great as a team. She said it was extra hard and that she wasn't sure if she wanted to do it again.

I told her how I wanted to be competing rather than watching and that if I could get fit enough, I wanted to try next year. She immediately perked up and said if I was going, she would too. So we made a deal and set it as a goal.

Sara came over after the workout to talk with me and gave me some advice about how the timeline could work in getting ready for next year. It was good advice. Now I am pumped about making that happen next year.

It is not about winning. It is about being able to compete and to be competent and fit enough to belong – even if it is in last place. If I don't embarrass myself, my partner or the box, I will be good!

The workout was deadlifts first – 5 sets of 5 reps every 2 ½ minutes. I was working off plates – lower to the ground than ever – rather than boxes. My form stayed good. I am almost ready to go to the ground. This is way cool.

I am able to tell where my muscles are, how my posture is, and if I am keeping tight. A year ago, I couldn't do any of those things because I had lost touch with my body. It is amazing to feel the difference.

Then we did 50-40-30-20-10 reps of kettle bell swings and sit ups with a time cap of 12 minutes. That is 300 reps in 12 minutes, and it is punishing. I was able to finish in 11:41. I think it is the first time I've broken 12 minutes!

The sense of continuing to progress, to grow, to change, to move better, to be stronger, to have more balance and stamina – it all feels so good. There is pride in how far I've come and a hunger to go much further. Thank you, CrossFit and thank you CFOC!

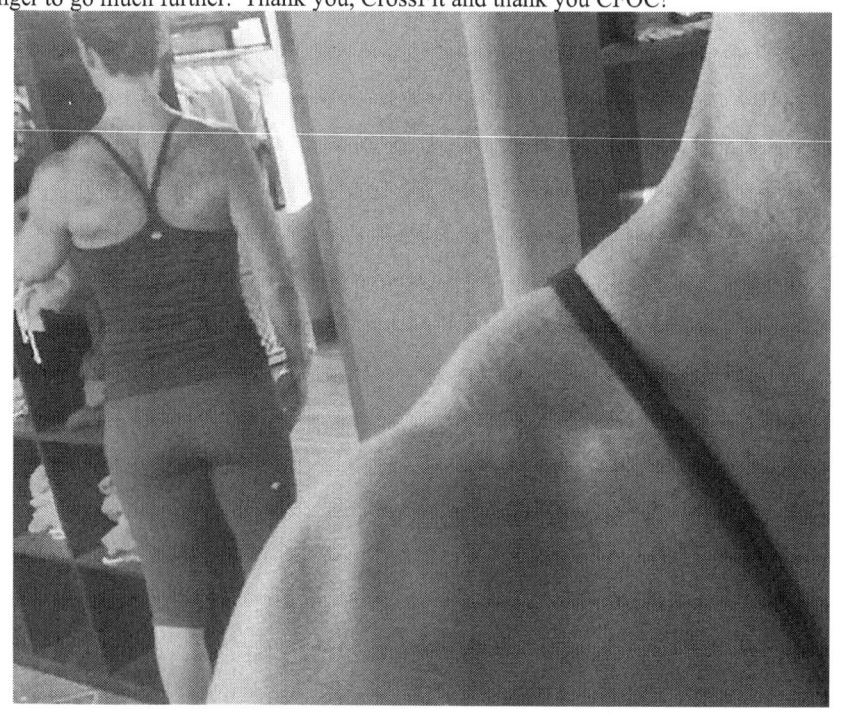

Jeannie Datria   48   RN

Jeannie is a very pleasant soft-spoken woman. She has a quiet intensity when she talks about crossfit that is powerful. As a younger woman she was active in volleyball and softball. She was a member of a regular gym and then Dani talked her into trying CFOC. She has been a member for 5 years.

Her initial experience was intense. She says it kicked her butt. She says that everybody was welcoming and non-judgmental. She wanted to get a good workout and to try something different. She certainly got that.

A few years ago, she hurt her back and had surgery. After 6 weeks she was able to ease back into her workout routine. She says that she always knew this is her family. It is a great experience.

She says that Jen sets the foundation. She is always there and never gives up on you. She is a special person and not just a business owner.

She says no matter what I am going through, this is where I need to be!

Today's workout follows the latest trend of being a killer. Dave is back and I thought he might want to partner, but he said he was going to take it easy and do it solo. Tiny walked through the door and pointed at me. I knew what that meant!

Brad went over the workout and we got set up. Tyler and Mike were close by and Dave was right next to us.

The workout went like this:
1-mile row – my goodness, what a way to start! Both partners had to do the mile.
75 alternate Dumb bell snatches – I am feeling good for these.
50 box stepovers with weight – Tiny and I pass on the weight, as doing a 20" box step overs are challenge enough
50 pull ups – again Tiny and I scale these doing ring pullups
800 m row – this is diabolical. An intense row in the middle of the workout. I am feeling this. Both partners must do 800 m.
50 pull ups – I have trouble catching my breath
50 box step overs – thank god for Tiny
75 Alt DB snatches – pure torture.
1-mile row – oh my!
The workout had a 40-minute time cap. Tiny and I finish in 34:50.

Tyler, Mike, Dave (who didn't take it easy), Tiny, Brad (who rowed with us), and I shouted encouragement and insults at each other throughout the workout. We pushed it hard. It looked so hard on paper and it *was* hard. But we crushed it and it felt so good. What a super way to start the day!

It is the Friday before Labor Day and it is a strange day at the Box. There are three coaches here at 9 AM plus Scott. One of the big warehouse doors has stuck at the top and there are issues trying to find someone to come fix it.

Brad decides to stay for the workout. Dani is coaching. It is one of those subtle little workouts that sneak up and kick your butt. A lot of my friends are here – Teri, Tiny, Gage, Rachel, and more – and there promises to be a lot of shared misery.

The first part is weightlifting...front squats or a barbell complex. I will do pistol squats (one-legged squats) while holding rings for balance. This is part of my program to equalize strength in both legs. I can't compensate doing only one leg at the time. And, these suckers are hard! It is 5 sets of 5 reps each leg every 2 minutes.

Teri and I have a nice chat while we are setting up for the metcon. She was in California getting her kids settled in for college. Lots of stress.

The metcon is 5 minutes of max reps of 10 deadlifts and 30 double-unders. I am doing jumping jacks for the double unders. I will start learning those shortly.

It is extremely hard. 1-minute rest.

5 minutes of hang power cleans and burpees to the barbell. Since I am doing burpees as described, it is hard and slow. 1-minute rest. Dani and Scott suggest that I use a little more height on the plates I'm using for the deadlifts as my back is not quite where it needs to be. I had gone lower again and it was too much.

5 minutes of 10 pull ups and 10 hand-release pushups – chest to the ground. This one is totally brutal. I am gasping for breath and had to do pushups from my knees for the last two sets.

Whoa! We sit around catching our breath and then start complaining about how hard it was. Soon, however we are all smiling and laughing. It is good to be alive.

Steve "Hoff" Hoffedtz   53   retired firefighter

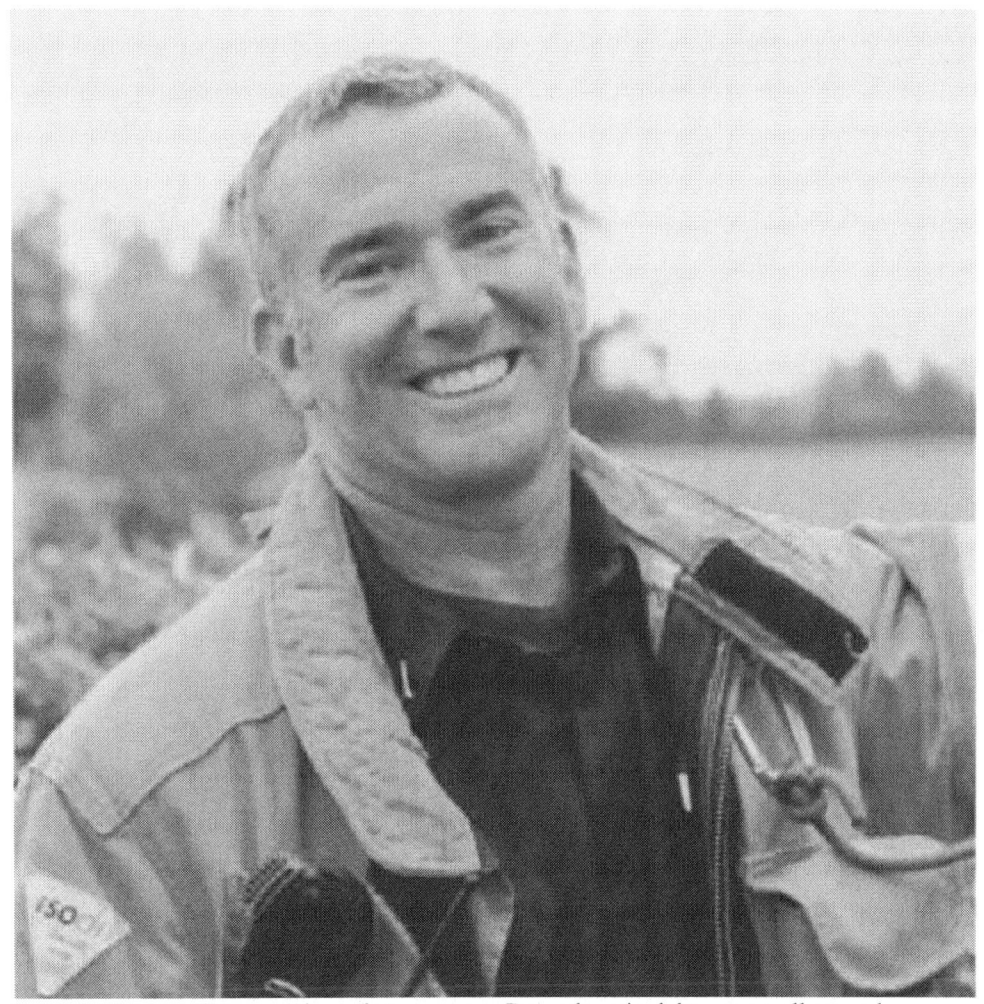

Hoff is a charismatic, energetic, and strong man. Recently retired, he was an all-around athlete since the second grade. He started weightlifting in high school and took part in many competitive sports. He did some running and started working out at Golds Gym in college and continued until 2014. He had some back issues and was concerned about what he heard about crossfit.

He had many friends already in the box and decided to give it a try…even though his first coach was a cop (he was smiling when he said it, but it was easy to see there is some heat in the rivalry between the firefighters and the law enforcement people). He said his back felt great. At first, he scaled most workouts. He came on Thursdays to get more coaching and progressed rapidly from there.

Hoff said that he felt a lot in common with most people at the box and he rapidly made some good friends. He sees many of his box friends socially for travel, golf, and other activities. He describes the relationships like this: I have a fire family and CFOC family. Both families are equally close.

He says he has lots of opportunities to make friends. What makes them special is for his fire family there is a common aspect of danger. For CFOC that aspect is pain. The teamwork aspect is the same.

He and his wife thought about moving, but asked themselves, "What are we going to do about CFOC?" They decided to stay.

He said that at CFOC everybody smiles. Everybody works out with friends. Everybody works hard – all in the same place!

He remarked that his stamina is unbelievable, that he feels fit both mentally and physically. He really enjoys the Hero and special workouts. They are always on his mind and he likes that they are particularly hard. Hoff shares big biceps like Don Wagoner and it probably is no coincidence that they are close friends. I think if I keep hanging out with them, I might gain some size in my "guns" ☺

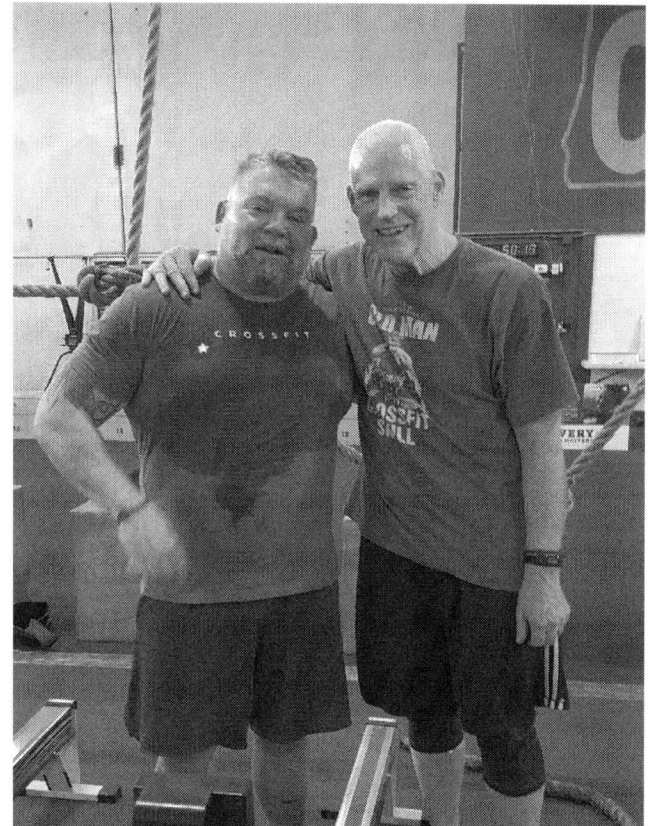

Steve Tiny Irwin

Tiny is a big man, with a big personality and a big heart. We work out together on the partner WODs on Wednesdays and I've had the chance to play golf with him and visit his home. He is a wonderful man.

Tiny never did sports except wrestling until high school. After high school he says the only physical activity he did regularly was bouncing at a San Diego bar. He became active later when he moved to the PNW and was active lifting – sometimes twice a day. He became friends with Josh (a coach at CFOC for quite a while) who encouraged him to do crossfit. He went 5 or six times to a box in Vancouver and did not like it at all.

Four years later, Josh told Tiny he had to try CFOC. That was 2, almost three, years ago. Tiny says he went to please Josh and met some good people. He was very intimidated. He is naturally strong, and he couldn't keep up. He was injured, and it forced him to change his mindset. He had to forget wanting to compete and to focus on form and execution. He felt accepted and was held accountable…which he says he needed.

Going to crossfit caused a rift at home. He lived in North Portland and the box is quite a distance from there. He says they managed to stay there another 8 months then found a house in Oregon City and moved the whole family. Then, out of nowhere, he lost his job. Because of CFOC they decided to stay in Oregon City.

His wife, Leah, started coming to the box and enjoyed it a lot. His two boys – 6 and 9 - came to the gym one Saturday to watch videos while Leah and Tiny worked out. They watched their parents working out and wanted to do what they were doing.

Marti started helping the kids lift and rope climb. Then more kids joined in and Jen, Ashley and Marti were leading a kids' class! Tiny says that sums up this community.

Tiny met Colin Wrede, a young youth minister at a local church, and "adopted" him. They work out together and hang out together a lot. Tiny has a bedroom for him in his house and has him over for dinner at least twice a week. Tiny says that he is really close to a couple of other people at the gym. He says that it is not just working out – it is a lifestyle. It is family. He says that it is the right mix of accountability, friendship, and the desire to be better.

Get there when you get there and do what you can do – that is Tiny's take on CFOC. Scott and Jen set the example; it is who they are. The coaches are great.

Tiny says it helps him be a better dad and husband. It is a special place.

Adam Durham   52   sales manager

Adam is, in chaos theory terms, a strange attractor. He disrupts flow. He attracts chaotic energy. He adds energy and impetus to the system. He is a force unto himself.

Adam is one of those people who do not have an off switch – or even a slow-down switch. As Ty commented to me while we were working out, Adam wants 4 years' experience as a crossfit athlete in 6 months. The only times he slows down at all is when he is injured. Even then, he tries to push through it.

He is good natured and a loving Dad to Beckham. However, he is a polarizing figure in the box. He has strongly held political views that he is not shy about expressing. He has an opinion about everything. He likes shouting encouragement during workouts. He is "that" guy.

Members either like him or dis-like him and stay away from him (but very politely – although some are straightforward with Adam and whatever he doesn't agree with bounces off him like he is wearing Kevlar).

I like Adam a lot. I don't agree with him and we have decided that is fine. I understand his need to be first, fast, on top of it, to exceed, to excel, and to push others to be that way as well. Adam is a "true believer" about crossfit and is constantly telling people how much he loves CFOC. He also offers motivational sayings and personal insights about parenting and many other topics. He doesn't understand why others don't express their love for CFOC the way he does.

Adam adds a much-needed dimension to CFOC. He adds diversity of opinion and outlook. He creates energy and awareness of differences. He gives spice to the mix. He provides a focal point for discharging negative energy in the system. As they say in the South, God bless him.

Today, as I was ruminating about the almost two years I've been a member of CFOC and thinking about my goals and where I stand, I came to a startling conclusion. I am still in the mode that caused me to realize I was out of touch with my body two years ago. I was thinking, "Todd, for 70 years old, you are in pretty good shape." Then I realized by putting it in those terms it allowed me to rationalize the belly fat that still bothers me and movements and form I am still struggling with and the lack of focus and discipline that allow me to cheat on my meal plan and shrug my shoulders about it.

Don't get me wrong, I am not saying that I need to be a perfectionist and to make unbelievable progress every month. What I am saying is that if I compare myself to others, I will not be focused on what *my* potential is and what *my* progress toward reaching that potential is.

I need to focus on what might be – *is* – possible for me. This is unchartered territory. I don't know how much strength, mobility, flexibility, and athletic movement I can still gain. I won't know unless I keep pushing my comfort zones and try to get better. Comparison is the road to mediocrity. It is the road to rationalization – *after all, I am over seventy.*

Bull puckey!

I am preparing for the summer games in Bend in August with the other Todd A. Weber as my partner and I am going to give it all that I can. All I can do is my best and that is what I plan to give to it.

It is so easy to slide into comfort zones and to stop pushing for excellence. For the older athlete there are all kinds of ways to slack off – just a bit. "Relax, you've earned it." "I hope I am in that kind of shape when I reach your age." "You are in better shape than most guys in their twenties or thirties." Which may or may not be true. What matters is am I in the best shape I can be? And the answer is resounding "NO!" I don't know the limits yet. I don't know when age will "catch up with me." My body feels better than it has in decades. It seems eager and able to keep pushing harder. If I stick to the advice Brad gave me about keeping it a progression of small steps and not a giant step that over-reaches my capacity, I will be fine.

Maybe I will find my limits. And maybe, there are no limits if I keep going one step after the other.

After contemplating what I just said about pushing it, I've had an interesting and eye-opening conversation with Brad about training cycles. He pointed out that you cannot go all-out every workout. You have to modulate the effort to the desired effect of the given workout and you have to factor in recovery.

An aging athlete must be much more aware of the need for recovery. I have been guilty of pushing too hard, too much, for too long. I am in a place right now of feeling run down and sore more than normal. The workouts for the past couple of weeks have been intense. I have pushed hard in the weightlifting portions as well.

As a result, I have a bunch of personal bests – and I am tired and not sleeping well.

Brad suggested going easy for a couple of weeks to recover. "Going easy" is a relative term. It is about an active recovery – not doing nothing. I will cut one workout a week and cut back to working with lighter weights rather than going for a PR every time ▯

When I am sleeping better and feel more fully recovered, I will start a new cycle with Brad to work on my weightlifting form and weights.

That means I will be doing one or two fewer strictly Crossfit workouts a week in order to sustain the weight work. It is exciting to be able to move forward with this work.

Today I had the first session working with Brad for the weightlifting meet. It was so much fun! It started with a good warm up, then using a PVC pipe about the length of a barbell, Brad had me working on form – mainly from the ground to just above the knee.

We are working on the snatch, which is a quick, technical, movement of the bar from the ground to overhead, with a wide straight-arm finish. You would think that making a bar go from your feet to overhead would be simple. It is not.

After Brad was satisfied with my movement from the ground to above the knee, we then started moving from the ground to the pull, which is a shrugging, pulling movement getting the bar moving quickly to the shoulder area. I may not be using the correct terms, but I hope you are getting the picture.

When Brad was satisfied (which is relative to my limitations in mobility,) we then worked on moving the PVC from the ground to overhead. Moving a PVC pipe that weighs maybe 3 pounds should be easy work. It is not. Just trying to get the correct movement over and over and over is exhausting. When Brad was satisfied, we took a little break while I got a 35-pound bar and two wooden discs that put the bar at the height it would be with weights on it.

Brad set his bar up with weight, then said we would alternate lifting. I would watch him lift, then I would lift. After each lift, Brad would have me critique my form in comparison to his. Then he would agree or make corrections. And we would do it again. It was so much fun. I was finally *feeling* where the bar was as I lifted. And I could tell what I was or wasn't doing. The word Brad gave me to concentrate on was "contact." He wanted me to make sure the bar contacted my shirt or body just at or above my hips as I pulled. Keeping the bar close stops it from moving forward which can cause the lifter to miss the lift.

After getting relatively good at 35#s I put 20#s on the bar for a total of 55#s, and we did it again. Brad lifted and then I lifted. Talking and critiquing after each set. I was really feeling good making so much progress.

Then we added 10 more pounds for a total of 65#. I have never snatched this much weight before. It went up easy! Absolutely amazing. We traded lifts again a couple of times. Brad said let's end on a high note and he added 5 more pounds for a total of 70#.

My first lift at 70# was a little rough as I ended with bent arms and pressed it out. For the snatch, that is not allowed. I went one more time and hit it perfectly. When my form and mechanics are right, it is almost as if the weight lifts itself. It is utterly amazing!

So, in one hour with Brad, I went from lifting PVC pipe to putting 70#s overhead. I was so happy. Just learning to get the bar off the floor with good form then completing the lifts with solid mechanics was an incredible feeling.

We will be working together once a week for now. It will be more often as the meet gets closer. Too cool for school!

I talked with Rick K. today at the gym. I only see Rick on Saturdays because he usually works out in the afternoon. He is a super nice guy and we usually have interesting conversations. Today we got talking about dogs and the 4th of July. He asked how my dog handled it and I said better than ever before with the help of a fan and CBD snacks.

We started talking about how my girl is doing after her brother died a few months ago. I told him that we both are still grieving and that she is doing better, but it is taking time. Her "brother" was a Landseer newfoundland 9 years old and she is 12 and a black newfy… which is quite old for a giant breed.

Rick has two dogs that are a bonded pair and he is concerned how they will handle it when one of them dies. So, it was a kind of downer conversation but typical of the depth and caring that takes place at the gym. People genuinely care about each other and go out of their way to offer help and comfort. I have never been part of a community that shows this much connection and concern. It is amazing.

Chapter Fifteen

Important!

This may be the most important thing I say in this book. It is so important that I have been struggling with how to say it without sounding pompous or arrogant or like a know-it-all. So, I will just put it out there.

Most things in our lives are out of our control. We certainly have no control over other people and their actions. There is little in our immediate or extended environment that we can control. We have no control over nature. We do not control the randomness of events and accidents. And we do not have or have limited control over our health and well-being.

That being said, we do have some control over our bodies, what we eat, how or if we exercise, how or if we read or continue to learn throughout life, how or if we socialize, and who and where we choose to spend our time.

Since there is so little we do control and the things we can control have such a huge potential impact on our health, fitness and well-being, it **seems obvious that we should put tremendous effort into our nutrition and fitness.**

IBM did a study a few years ago concerning cardiac surgeons and cardiologists and their patients who had a major cardiac event. IBM asked the physicians how many of their patients changed after having "the conversation" after surgery with the family present. It goes like this: Mr. Smith (it is a male a large percentage of the time), you were lucky this time. We got to the issue before major damage occurred and were able to repair it. However, you need to know that if you do not change the way you are living, it will happen again, and the odds are you will die.

Do you understand what I am saying Mr. Smith – Mrs. Smith and little Smiths? You will die if you do not change your diet and exercise habits!

IBM asked the physicians how many of the patients change. The answer was 1 in 9. One out of nine people who were told that it was **change or die** decided to change. **1 in 9!!**

Do you understand how absurd that is?

I am saying the same thing here: no matter how old you may be, no matter your health condition, no matter your fitness level, you can and must change! You may not have total control of the situation, but you can make changes that will impact your health and fitness and quality of life.

And, there is only one day you have control over to start changing and that is **today!**

That is it. Today – now – is all we can control. This instant, right now, we can change. Not think about it. Not plan it. Not talk it over. Not start next week. Not do some research. Not consider the options. Now! Take action! Intention does not count. It is intention put into action that gets results. Start right now!

How you age, your fitness level, your likelihood of chronic lifestyle diseases, your quality of life, all depend on the choice you make right now. It is that simple. And it is that hard.

When I was younger, I thought I was bulletproof. I took my health and fitness for granted. I didn't think about long-term consequences of my diet and exercise and other choices I was making every day. Then, I became even more complacent in my 40s, 50, and 60s. Sure, I had put on some pounds and couldn't move the way I used to. But compared to other people my age, I was doing pretty well.

I was really fooling myself and avoiding looking at the truth. Until I was lucky enough to wake up.

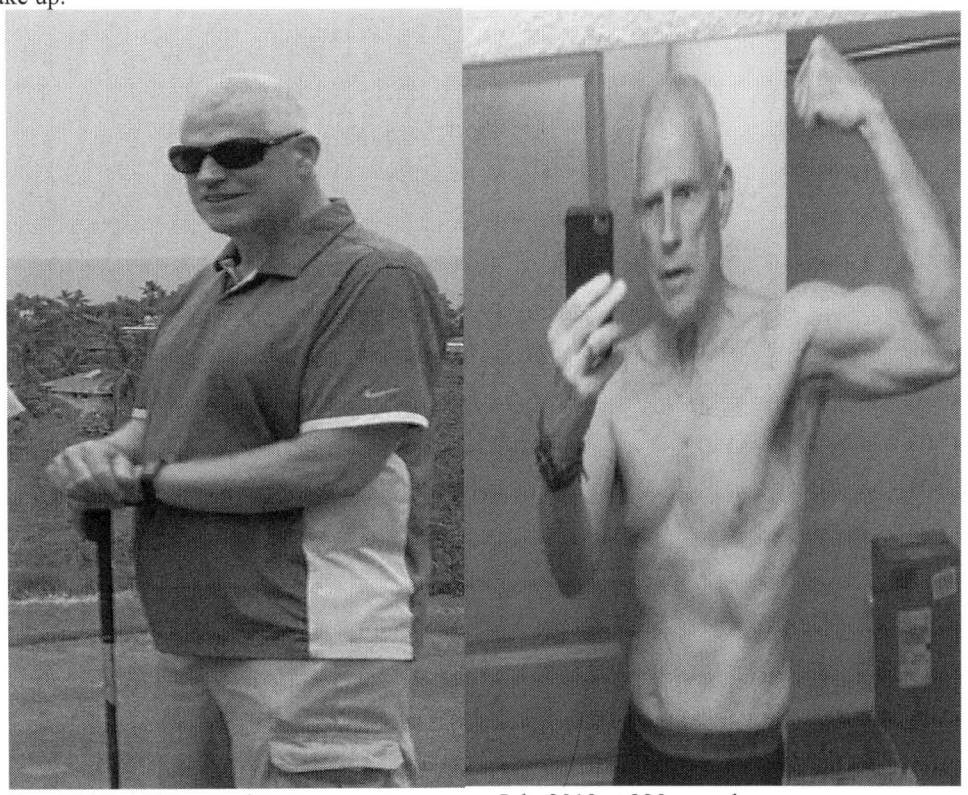

June 2017 at 275 pounds   July 2019 at 220 pounds

The difference is more than just the weight. My body composition is different. I can move so much better. I have mobility and flexibility. I have regained strength. I eat better. I have more energy. My posture is better. And, I am happier.

This is a gift that we can give ourselves if only we choose to act today!

Please make good choices right now. Don't wait until things are more under control – they never are. Don't wait until your finances are better – how expensive is poor health? Don't wait until the kids are older – set an example for them now.

This is something you can do right now that will impact the rest of your life.

Man, I wish I could be with you right now to convince you. Take the plunge and figure it out later.

OK, I will get out from behind my pulpit.

I did a lifting workout with Brad today. There is something about the lifts that makes me feel like a kid. I get excited and I get nervous and I get so pumped up when I complete a good lift. There is a satisfaction in learning and executing a technical and strenuous movement that is totally engrossing. You can't be anywhere else. You must be totally present and it is captivating.

Brad had to slow me down. Then he had to say enough is enough. We lifted for an hour. I felt like I could keep going for a long time. I am home and glad Brad stopped us. My traps are sore, my grip and all the muscles supporting my grip are sore. My lats are tight. And I know I will be feeling other muscles later. It sure feels good.

Colin Wrede 30yrs old.   Youth Pastor

Colin grew up playing sports. He loved basketball and football. He found CrossFit in Gresham, where he was working at a church. After 2 yrs, he got a new position as a youth pastor at a church in Canby and found CFOC. He said he was pretty intimidated the first few times at CFOC. Then he met a couple of guys who were really kind. He was impressed with the coaching and the support from the community.

He says that CrossFit respects nobody – it doesn't matter who you are, it humbles everyone! He likes the healthy competition and that everyone is on the journey to fitness. He learns a lot that carries over to his job. He says it is the uniqueness of the community, the accountability/suffering together, the commitment to keep coming – it pushes him to be better in every aspect of his life.

Colin is a happy soul who attracts people to his open acceptance. He says it is like CrossFit – it takes me where I am and helps me get better and better every day. It builds mental toughness and exposes weaknesses. It is what I want to do with my life.

He says you have to take the risks in order to reap the benefits and rewards. He says great things happen when you do the best you can with a bunch of other people doing their best.

In talking about crossfit, it is easy to see it as a black or white, yes or no, good or bad decision. Folks tend to go all in – "drink the Kool aid" - when starting with a box. However, I think it is important to note that many people do crossfit their own way.

It is true that I advocate for the older athlete to be active at an intense level at least 5 times a week. But that does not mean "all out" 5 times a week. Many knowledgeable sports and fitness experts promote a pattern of cycling in and out of different levels of intensity throughout the year, throughout the month, and even throughout the week.

As noted, aging athletes need more recovery time, more careful nutrition and more careful workout planning to get the most benefit from crossfit. You cannot go all out all the time. Neither can you go easy all the time.

Crossfit recommends a 5-day cycle with two rest days during the week. For an aging athlete, a four-on three-off pattern may be more beneficial. That does not mean the "off" days are total rest days. It means that there is active recovery during those days which could mean doing mobility and flexibility, or trying a new sport, or doing enjoyable hiking or biking or skating or skiing or doing accessory work on muscle groups not necessarily targeted during crossfit.

The aging athlete has concerns that may or may not be important to younger athletes. One major concern is muscle imbalances. Off days are good for working on these imbalances.

Another major concern for aging athletes is balance. Balance is crucial as we age in order to lessen the chance of falling – which is also why weight bearing exercise is so important. Off days are also a good time to work on those issues.

Check with the coaches at your box to determine what might be the best approach for you. It will change over time as your body gets fitter and stronger. Things will also change as you master movements and form. The exact mix of workouts and days will be a moving target. And it will help build your awareness as you listen to your body.

When I first heard "listen to your body" I thought "Well duh! Who doesn't listen to their body?" Then I began to realize it is different for athletes – in particular, aging athletes. In many cases we have lost touch with how to activate certain muscles or how to feel them when they are active. We may have lost touch with the small stabilizing muscles in the shoulders, hips, knees, and ankles. We may be comfortable with the movements that we habituated from years of moving only one way or one direction. And, we may feel uncomfortable with other movements or unable to do them.

Learning to "feel" these muscles again and then how to strengthen and activate them is important in getting fitter. And it puts stress on the central nervous system as we learn how to do it. It seems to be only common sense, but it is so important to be aware of.

Much of the benefit of fitness for the aging athlete is about gaining or re-gaining self-awareness. I think it is one of the reasons that doing crossfit is so much fun. Like when we were kids, we are learning (or re-learning) movements and form and strength and gaining the awareness in how to do the movements better or faster or stronger. It is fun! It is challenging! It pushes our limits. It gets us out of our comfort zones. It is how we keep growing.

Mike Myers   47 years old.   Commercial Airline Pilot

"Captain Mike" is a solidly built, consistent athlete. As you might expect from his profession, he is committed and focused. He grew up playing soccer, running, and doing triathlons. He found crossfit in Lake Oswego and was a member there for 5 years.

He liked it so much that he bought crossfit equipment for his garage and worked out at home. After one year of that, he wanted to increase the intensity of his workouts and joined CFOC.

He says that it is always super friendly. There is always someone he knows to workout with.

Mike talks about crossfit being totally in the moment. He says his life now is about spending lots of time feeling particularly good! He says the special workouts are a gut check for him. They are important in that they bring the box together and make him want to be better as a human being.

"There is joy in feeling healthy," according to Mike. He likes how it keeps him motivated.

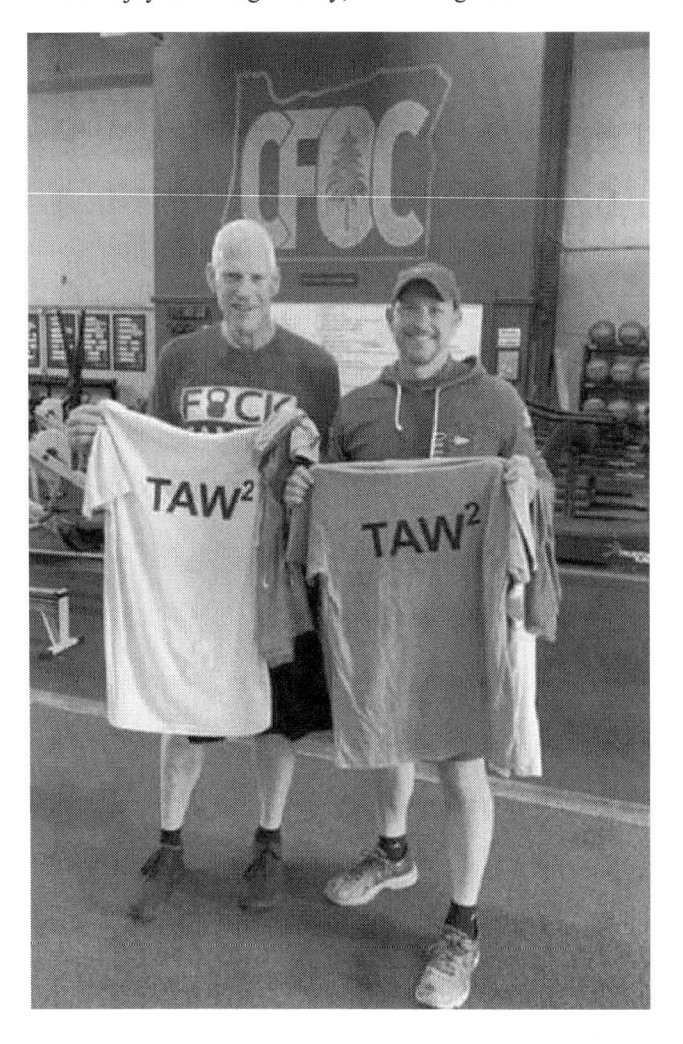

Summer is an interesting time in the box. There are many people preparing for competitions – like me for the first time. It is exciting and creating anxiety at the same time. I do not want to let my friends or my partner down, so I am taking the preparation seriously.

I get to see and workout with folks that I don't normally see. There is an intensity that is ratcheted up a notch or two. There is a lot of fun and socializing. And there is a lot more running in the workouts because the weather is good.

We always have the option to row instead of run, but I have been trying to consistently run as it stresses my body differently and is harder than rowing for me. I am slow…really slow. But I am faster than I was last year. I am trying to make slow, but consistent progress.

Along with the weightlifting workouts I am doing with Brad, I feel my body being strained in different ways and causing growth and increasing strength in ways I haven't felt before.

My traps are getting stronger from the "pulls" in the snatch and clean & jerk lifts. Most of the energy comes from the legs (I hear Brad's voice saying "Lift with your legs!), but the pull guides and balances the weight as the lifter settles under it.

My core is getting stronger as I am working on opening my thoracic spine to get my shoulders and arms back to receive the weight over my head. My whole core is stronger as I tighten it when preparing to explode into the lift.

As an aging athlete, getting the mobility to be able to have good form in the lifts is important. And, as Brad tells me, I may never have perfect form, but I will have workable form that is safe and consistent.

I have so much fun working on the lifts. I had no idea how technical and precise Olympic lifting is. One little thing that is off by a quarter of an inch can throw the whole lift off. It is about trying to get a very consistent and reliable process that produces good lifts every time. That takes practice, practice, practice and feedback to catch the little changes needed in order to improve. It is hard and oh so much fun!

Today I read an article online from a Medical Journal that talked about a drop of 32% in the chance of having dementia for people who live a healthy lifestyle. I thought to myself, "Well, duh!" Much of the current research on aging is centered on reducing the chance of chronic lifestyle diseases: cancer, arthritis, diabetes, heart disease, Alzheimer's Disease, and more. The overwhelming consensus is that a healthy lifestyle – exercise and clean nutrition – will lower the chance of having these diseases dramatically.

It is like we discussed earlier; if you knew for sure that exercise and clean eating would increase your odds of leading a quality life, why wouldn't you do it? It is a "no brainer," right?

And, as we talked about, only 11% of people who had a serious heart incident subsequently change their lifestyle.

Why? Why is it so hard to change? Why would we even hesitate to make the necessary changes?

From the research it seems that the "comfort zone" is so attractive and so addictive that we cannot give it up – even if it kills us.

The known – even the obviously unhealthy known – is more attractive than the unknown. And because of that, we have serious problems making necessary changes.

Making gradual, step-by-step changes clearly doesn't work. The research shows over and over again that people will backtrack very quickly from that type of change. So, what does work? The key is to change BIG quickly.

It is called "**Punctuated Equilibrium.**"

You disrupt your current lifestyle as much as you can and change your exercise and eating drastically. You hit it big and hard! You pile up as much success as quickly as you can. You throw all the old food out. You give the TV away. You walk everywhere. Or ride your bike. You do Crossfit 5-6 days a week. You eat clean.

After two or three weeks when you are noticing big changes, but the old siren song of the couch and potato chips is calling your name, you look for help, support and structure.

You talk to your coaches at Crossfit to get ideas about the best food plans that are sustainable. You talk to the friends you have gained at Crossfit to see how they do it and what kind of support they have found. You hang around people who have the same kind of goals you have and who are making the same kind of changes. You do the things that support and enhance your efforts.

And, **you show up every day at the box,** no matter what.

It is a process, not an event. It takes time and effort. Every day you will make changes. Every day you will get stronger. Every day your body will get healthier. Just 1% difference every week, will mean a 50% change in a year! That is worth the effort, isn't it?

People fail because they start making excuses to not show up. I'm too busy or its too expensive. Good health is too expensive? Try the cost of poor health for a comparison. No matter how you feel and or what you are thinking, show up every day! Every damn day. Your friends at the box will support you and help you. They are working on the same lifestyle you are. They have been through or are going through the same things you are. They want you to succeed just as you want them to.

How do you think you will feel later if you don't make the changes you know you should? How will you feel when you start or increase having the health issues you could have avoided or made less debilitating?

This is about your body, your health, your fitness. It is one of the few things that you have control over to some extent. And if you fail to make changes that you could have, and it results in a poorer quality of life – what then?

I am begging you. Do it! Don't have regrets about what could have been. It is not just your life that is influenced by your changes. It is your kids and grandkids and friends and neighbors and co-workers and others at the box and more. You can be a symbol of what is possible. It is not about being perfect. It is about making little changes every day. Doable changes. Every day.

Don't take my word for it. Go to a Crossfit box and talk to people there about their lives and the changes that have occurred. Ask questions. Look around. If it doesn't feel right, find another box. Then get to work!

Erin McCart   48 years old   direct product management and marketing

    Erin is an incredible athlete. He is strong, agile, and focused. He is also asthmatic. He says that Jen and Scott helped research his needs as an athlete and help keep him on track.
    His nutrition has changed dramatically. He schedules crossfit as part of his workday. He found after about six months that he had a need to be perfect. He got upset with himself. His friends and coaches helped him realize that it is the process and not comparing himself with others that is what it is about.
    He says he wants to return the favor by helping others. His self-confidence has grown tremendously. He is more successful at his work. He says that it is humbling to be part of crossfit and to realize that there is still so much more fitness to gain and things to learn.
    He has learned that crossfit is his retreat from daily life. It is his happy place! It is OK to do 80% or 90% sometimes… and to enjoy the process.

    The community seems to be going through a change in dynamics currently. Scott is back on the road working to secure funding to buy a building, so he is not seen much in the box. Jen is working the afternoon classes. Brad is working more over-time, so he is not coaching as much.
    There are underground and not so underground mumblings about some members' kids' behavior and other members social behavior. 18 teams are preparing for the Summer Games in Bend. Some of the membership is dealing with family cancer problems.
    It is not uncommon for a tightknit group like this to go through adjustments occasionally. I don't know the whole history of the box and so I don't know if this has happened before. My guess is that it has.
    It will take a while for it all to shake out. Then we'll see what has changed. Meanwhile, we are working out, having fun, pushing and helping each other and enjoying the nice Summer.

Steve Hohensee   50 yrs old   Clackamas County Sheriff

    Steve is a soft-spoken man who is immensely strong. He has a quiet confidence and demeanor that befits his position as a deputy sheriff.
    Steve was active in sports in HS with football and wrestling. He went on to play one year of football at Lewis & Clark College. He then did 8 years of active duty in the Army before becoming a deputy sheriff.
    From being active in sports, he fell in love with weightlifting. He said his initial experience at crossfit was unlike anything else he has experienced. People were nice and cautioned him not to compare himself to other athletes in the box. But his competitive nature came out and he had to learn to moderate his work at the beginning.
    Some workouts can be really challenging, and they are always different, which he really enjoys.
    He says that no one judges. He sees people he works with and he socializes with others. His major battle is in showing up. He says if he forces himself to come, it works. Everyone is welcoming and open.
    He likes that everyone has common goals, that it is safe to be himself, and that it feels like family.

Before the workout this morning, I was talking with Teri and her daughter Daylin. I was complaining about being sore and tired and not really wanting to do the workout. Then I stopped myself and said to Teri, but that isn't the kind of people we are, is it?

We understand that today is all we have, and we can't even guarantee that. Nothing is promised. This instant is all there is. We make it what it is. It is about our relationships – right here and right now. It is about our attitude – right here and right now. It is about who we choose to be in this moment.

Teri and Daylin were smiling, saying that's why we like you Dr. Todd. You always turn things around and find the sunlight and the positive. I smiled back and said – I remind myself almost every day what a gift it is!

The workout was two separate components that were hard, but not a butt kicker. It was worth showing up. And it reminded me that being here is half the battle.

Kyle Bangs   27   Chiropractor

Dr. Kyle is a tremendously fit young man. He has a positive attitude and is willing to help at a moment's notice.

His office was right next to – almost embedded in – CFOC. Then he and his partner found a larger space and moved. Kyle was highly active in sports and did intramurals in college. He majored in kinesiology and then went on the chiropractor school.

Kyle started Crossfit in Vancouver then found CFOC when he came to practice in Oregon City. His initial experience was intense, he said. Always being pushed. Feeling intimidated. But the atmosphere was great, and the support was tremendous. The workouts were horrible, but he always felt great afterward.

He made great friends and does many activities with them outside the box. He says the relationships are special. Really close, not just gym buddies. Jen is always giving.

Kyle says that exercise makes you a better person – it effects your whole life.

It is the relationships that create such a special community at crossfit. For the older athlete, the special bonds formed are a true gift. If we are to be truly aware and truly present to this moment – this relationship – this experience, we must let go of the past and not look into the future. Now is what we have. Part of the awareness of now for the ageless athlete is the acceptance and understanding of death.

Death is the punctuation that provides meaning to our lives. If we had eternity, this moment and the next and the next would hold no special meaning. Knowing this moment may be our last provides the sweet experience of an ending. We can bring ferocious attention to now because it is all we have.

Fitness, health, the experiences of growing and changing and still having room to increase our potential and capacities is magical for the ageless athlete. We can be present – because we are practicing everyday with our fitness. We can be present to our pain and suffering and to our joy and wellness that our fitness practice provides. And it adds an element of closeness to every relationship we have. We can reach out and connect as a whole being and bring to our relationships our total self.

This is not something we may have considered when we started our fitness journey. However, it is a benefit that is full of grace.

Today was a good day! I achieved a PR I'd been planning on for quite a while as a goal. It took longer than I expected because I had to start squatting again from the beginning when I had the strength imbalance issues in my hips.

Once I was able to do a proper squat, it still took time to build the strength equally and to strengthen the stabilizer muscles in my legs, butt, hips, and back.

Then, not too long ago, it started to accelerate. I was gaining strength quickly and starting to squat with more "authority." Today I was able to back squat 200# three times!

It was incredible. My friends celebrated with me. It is still giving me a smile as I think about it.

What made it even more incredible was a conversation I had with a friend right after this morning's workout. He asked me what I thought was an odd question at first. He asked if I hung out with people my own age. After I thought about it, I answered that other than Dave, my workout partner at CFOC, I did not. He asked why.

I said that I don't know many people my age who have the energy, the vitality, the initiative to go after life with a gusto the way I want to. The people at crossfit do, and not many others that I know.

So, that is who I hang with.

He said that he understood. He told me he had a conversation with a 70 yr old man the previous evening. The conversation got on to fitness and he asked the man why he didn't work out and stay active. The man said that he was too old for that and he was "past" it.

It made me so sad – and so mad – to hear this. Many folks give up on life and health and fitness even though there is so much to gain. No matter a person's condition and health status, fitness and healthy eating can improve the quality of life. PERIOD!

Yes, it takes work. Yes, it takes discipline. Yes, it takes focus. But the benefits are so incredible.

I didn't want to be "that guy." The one nobody wants to sit next to on the plane. So, I took action. There is nothing special about me. I am not some amazing human specimen. I started working out and eating clean. And I kept doing it every day. And I got results. I kept doing it every day. And, now over 2 years later, I am still growing stronger and gaining capacity and feeling better. How can this not be worth it? How can it not be the obvious choice? I don't get it.

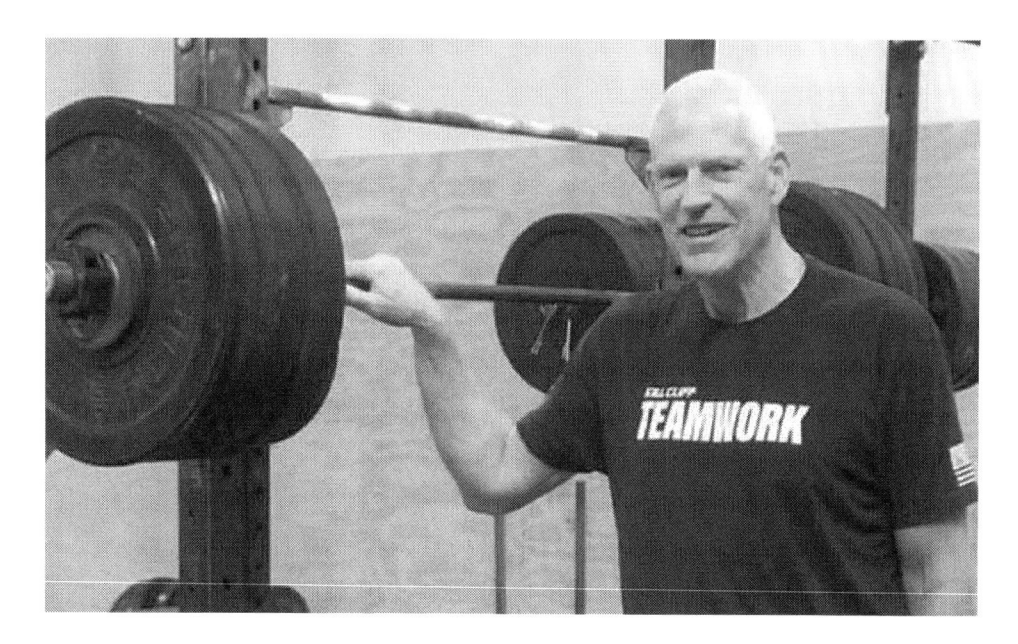

I don't know how to make it any clearer or more compelling that things can be better! It is not a false hope or claim. Do the work and you will get results. Eat clean and your health will improve.

Oh man, it is so frustrating to hear about conversations like that.

Today I was talking with a couple of ladies at the box about yesterday's workout. We were discussing how difficult it was and compared it to a couple of other workouts this week. It was like a hundred other post-workout conversations at the box.

Driving home, I realized something. It was a difficult workout, there is no doubt about that. But it was not as difficult as it should have been for me. I got a good sweat and I am sure I benefited from the work. I did not get outside my comfort zone, however.

The workout was ten 4-minute rounds of sand-bag work, toes-to-bars and burpees to a target, max airdynne calories, and 1-minute rest. A total of 40 minutes. Hard – very hard – and not hard enough for me.

I chose a sandbag weight that was too easy. The toes-to-bars and burpees were good. And I could have pushed the airdynne calories much harder as there was a minute to rest before starting the sandbags again.

I remember my commitment to get the most out of my workouts. Not going all out every workout but making each workout count and trying to be on the edge of my capabilities with a reasonable -and smart – plan for recovery.

I could have pushed this workout much harder. I had an active recovery day planned for the next day. It was work I could do without much concern for safety. I blew it.

I promised myself today to try to be more aware of when I can push hard…of when I can get to the edge of comfort…of when I can make the hard choice. I want to be able to continue to progress. That is important to me. I need to build better awareness of when I am "safe" and when I can go for it.

This past weekend I was in Bend OR for a crossfit competition called "The Best of the West." It is put on by Crossfit Oregon, a box in Bend. It attracts hundreds of athletes, supporters, and families for two days of competition. It is my first crossfit competition.

I was excited and nervous to take part. CFOC had 18 teams of two people – same sex- in different categories. My partner (Todd A. Weber) and I were competing in the scaled men's category. We were the oldest competitors (or I was) by far.

It was so challenging and so fun. It was amazing. The last event for us on Sunday – since we did not make the finals – was 5 rounds of 400m run and DT. DT is 12 deadlifts, 9 hang power cleans, and 6 shoulder to overheads. The weight was 95 pounds, which is heavy for scaled. I was able to do the deadlifts and cleans, but not the overheads, so Todd had to do those.

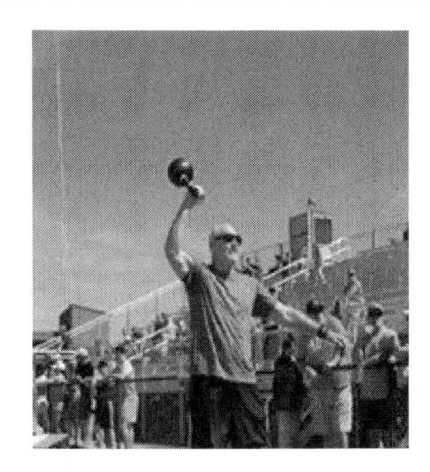

I ran first, then we split the reps, then Todd ran, and so on. We were cheered by a good-sized crowd and by the folks from CFOC. I ran the last 400m and as time ran out, I was about 2/3 done. All the competitors from CFOC and many from other teams ran out on the track to finish the final meters with me. The crowd was cheering, I was crying, and the announcer was saying something about if a 70 yr old athlete could do this, so could anyone. It was totally amazing.

People came up to high-five me and talk to me. It happened all weekend long, but particularly after that event. It was so gratifying. And it was so embarrassing.

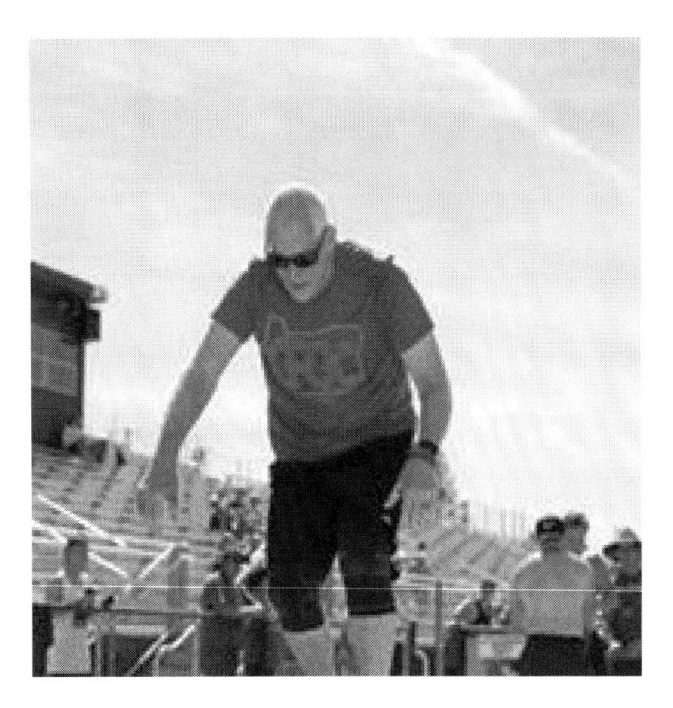

I was talking to Jay, my physical therapist, the next day about why I felt embarrassed. There is nothing special about me. I am not a world class athlete. I am a regular guy who decided to do Crossfit because I was tired of being tired, and fat, and slow, and feeling old. Anyone my age could do it.

Jay said, "But they don't do it, do they?" He said that I am an example and an inspiration for people who think they can't do it for whatever reasons. I can help lead the way.

He said, "Look at you!" Your posture is amazing. You are lean and strong. You move well. And, this is the most important, you are consistent and focused.

He said that I would be amazed with how many people come to him for treatment and who did not do the exercises and stretches he suggests. He said that people are looking for the easy way out… a pill, a one-time appointment, something to read. You, on the other hand, jump right into the process and work at it. I can tell how you improve from appointment to appointment. I love working with you.

And that is why you have benefitted so much from Crossfit. You do the work.

One of the insights I gained from doing the competition was that I will push myself extra hard – beyond what I think is possible – in order to not let my partner down. I did things I didn't think I had the capacity for and I set a couple of personal records. It was not about beating other teams. It was about seeing where my limits were and trying to exceed them.

And because of that, I realize that I still have areas -many areas – where I can grow, get better, get stronger, move better, learn new movements, build more endurance, build more speed --- basically continue to become a better athlete. And, a better person.

I don't think I am close to my potential. I don't know what my potential is, but I intend to try to keep moving toward it. It is so exciting to realize that there is so much more to gain. And there is so much more to share. There is no doubt that I am getting younger every day!

Chapter Sixteen

Since the competition I have been focused on Olympic lifting in preparation for my first weightlifting meet. Brad, Eddie, Nate, Sara and a few others are meeting before or after regular workouts to focus on lifting. I am learning so much and improving tremendously.

Brad is an exceptionally good coach. He is enthusiastic, passionate, and fun. I am learning the technical details and form for the two Olympic lifts: the snatch and the clean and jerk. Both lifts are done regularly during WODs. However, the preparation is different for the meet. The standards for a successful lift are stricter and Brad is emphasizing correct form in every aspect of the lifts.

I had no idea how exact and detailed each movement must be. I am improving by leaps and bounds and it is helping my crossfit performance as well.

We compete in 5 weeks. It is the final preparation phase of determining the weights to start with and go up with. Each lift has three attempts. The best lift of the three is added to the best of the other lift for a total weight. Six total lifts. Bam! It is much different than a crossfit competition. I am excited to see what happens when I am in front of a crowd. Freeze or lift? I am sure I am going to make that lift.

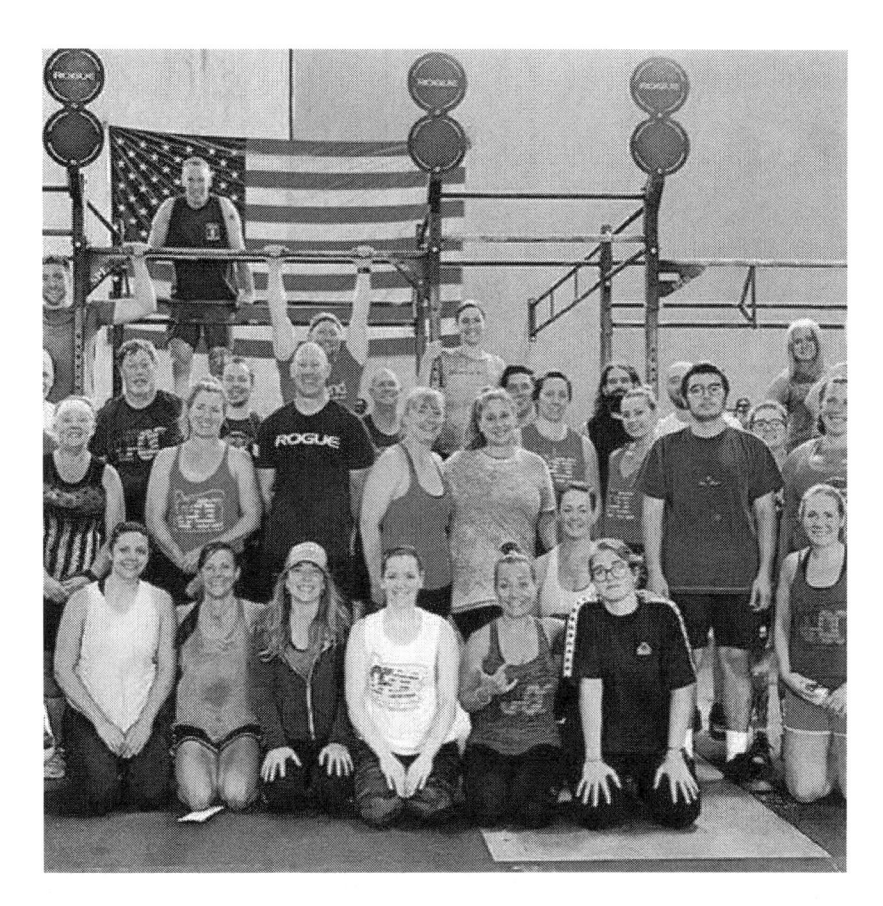

The past few weeks have been busy at the box. There are many families who have people with cancer. The box has been supporting many directly and indirectly through workouts, t-shirt sales, and direct donations. It is amazing to see the members come together to do what they can to help each other.

I am blown away by the love and support that is given. It makes me proud to be a member of this box.

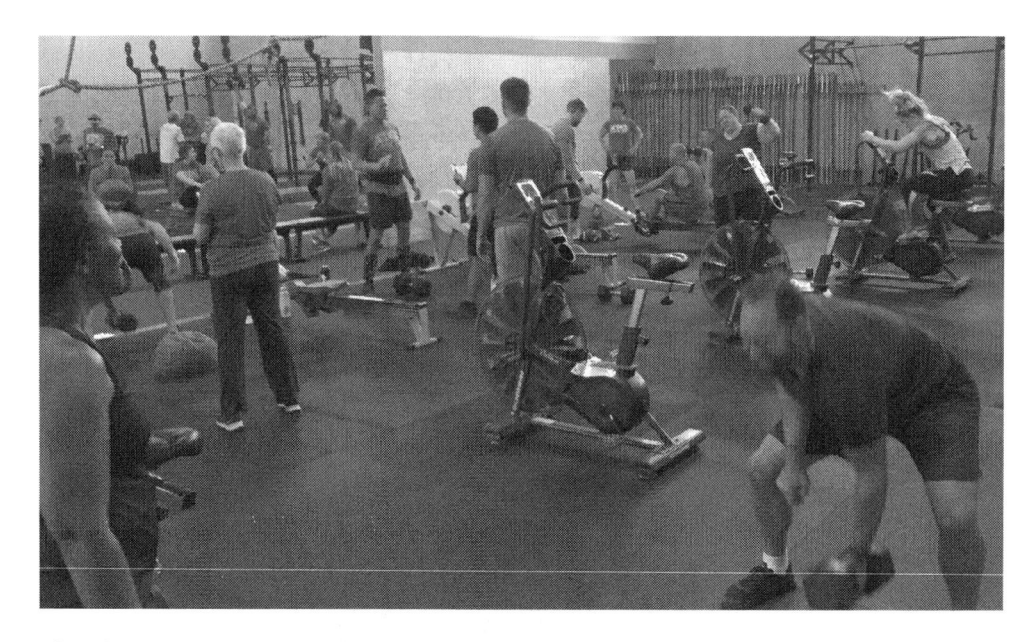

There is a magic moment in lifting when all the elements of the lift come together. The form is good. The power is good. The mind is right. And then, it is like the weight lifts itself. Then I think, "I've got it! I finally figured it out." And the very next lift is a mess.

I am having so much fun learning to lift correctly. It can be frustrating when it seems like I've forgotten everything I've been practicing. And then magic happens. Then I feel like I can make every lift.

The competition is four weeks away. I am working to establish what my opening lifts will be with Brad. My goal is to get the qualifying total for my age group and weight category which is 91 Kilograms. If I can get that total, then I can enter national meets.

Lifting makes me feel like a kid again on the playground. I'm following the big kids, trying to do what they can do. When I can do it, it is so exciting and fun. And the process itself is fun!

I'm getting to know Brad, Eddie, Sara and Nate so much better. We lift as a group at least once a week and sometimes more. There is energy and happiness and connection. I have a sense of abiding joy from these sessions.

I know that whether I do well in Seattle or not it will not matter in terms of my satisfaction.

The meet in Seattle was amazing. The people were supportive, encouraging, welcoming, and fun! Ex-Olympians, Masters World Champions, Pan Am Champions, National Champions all were present and were warm and gracious people.

I lifted well, but did not get a total as my snatches were not quite up to technical standards. My clean and jerk was good- I made two out of three lifts and received a silver medal in my age and weight category. I also achieved an Oregon State Record for my lifts. Of course, there probably wasn't an existing record before, but it is still pretty cool. I know that I will do much better in the future and I am looking forward to lifting in many more meets.

Brad is a proud coach and lifter. He received three silver medals in his category.

It was amazing to see athletes in the 90s, 80s, 70s, 60s all the way down to 35 who were erect with an athletic posture, moving well, and able to lift a lot of weight. It made me so happy that I am on this path.

It showed me that the intense exercise that is necessary for turning on the repair and growth function in the cells is not limited to cross fit or functional fitness. Many of the lifters had a cross fit background, but most came from lifting only. As one older lifter told me, it is the key to the fountain of youth.

I am trying to work closer to the edge of my capacity. Not all the time and not in every workout, but enough to trigger the growth and repair mechanisms more.

I want to continue to grow and change at a pace that is as close to my potential as possible. It means balancing and managing my intensity and effort with my recovery and sleep more carefully. I am measuring my resting heart rate (RHR), my heart rate variability (HRV), and my sleep to determine my state of recovery. I use a device called Whoop. It is a little pricey, but the information is very useful.

RHR is used a general marker for overall health. It can show when a person is getting run down or sick and needs more rest. HRV measures a different part of the heartbeat. Let's take a heart rate of 60 beats a minute. The time between each beat is not exactly one second each time. It varies based on several factors, the most important for athletes is showing how ready the heart is for heavy work. The greater the variability, the more ready the heart is.

And last is measuring sleep. The myth is that older athletes need less sleep as they get older. That could not be further from the truth. Sleep is necessary for the repair and restore functions to take place in the cells. Good nutrition plays a role here as well. The Whoop measures sleep cycles, disturbances, respiratory rate, circadian rhythm, and more.

Added together, the values provide a clear picture of my readiness for heavy and intense work. Conversely it shows when I need to back off to get some rest and recovery. These are especially useful tools for the aging athlete to make sure that they get the most out of their workouts and are not overtraining.

What an amazing couple of weeks. I received feedback from my doctor, who addressed me as the "healthiest and fittest 70-year-old I know." My PT told me I am an inspiration and example for him and many others who are watching my journey. A couple of members of CFOC came up to me out of the blue to say how much they admire me and hope they will be able to work as hard as I do when they are older.

I am humbled and inspired by these comments. I feel so grateful for finding this lifestyle. I feel so good having this community as support, accountability partners, inspiration, friends, and family. I am in awe of how hard my crossfit friends work, how they help each other, how they reach out to support the community, and how generous they are in cheering and encouraging others to do their best.

I am honored to be coached so well and to have made a great friend in the process.

I am so proud to be a member of CFOC.

I hope you find a home as I have. I hope you embrace the fitness lifestyle and live a long and quality life. All my best.

The Ageless Athlete

The keys to becoming an Ageless Athlete seem clear:

Workout intensely daily – or at least 5 times a week.

Eat "clean."

Get plenty of sleep.

Be part of a community that supports and encourages you.

Moderate stress through mediation, relaxation techniques, and/or breathing exercises.

Build self-awareness and awareness of others.

Stay in the moment.

Keeping a regimen that will result in being an Ageless Athlete is hard. It requires focus, discipline, commitment, and persistence. It is not an "easy fix" or short-term solution. It is a lifestyle.

But, look at all the benefits!

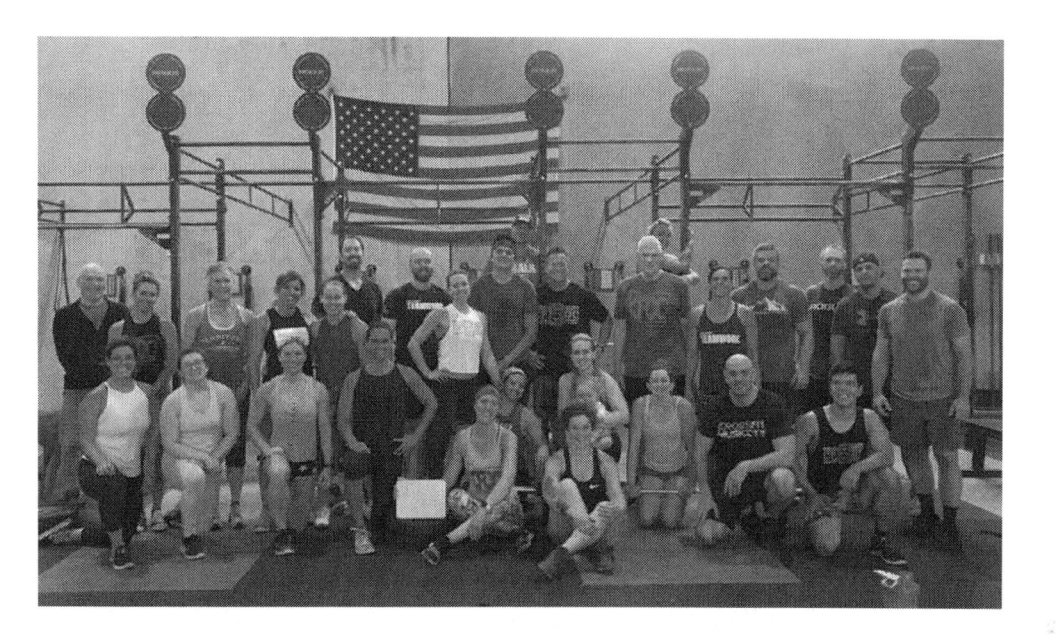

COVID-19

Coronavirus has changed many things, hasn't it? But one thing it hasn't changed – in fact it has reinforced it – is the need for older folks to get fit and stay fit. One of the most vulnerable populations in the pandemic are folks over 60. In particular, older folks with some kind of chronic condition are most likely to catch it and to die from it.

I am willing to bet when the statistics are analyzed that older folks who were fit were one of the least impacted groups. The reasons are pretty clear: a fit person's immune system is in better shape; in general, fit people eat healthier; fit people have a supportive community (even in social distancing); and fit people are less likely to suffer from depression, diabetes, heart disease and other chronic conditions that make a person more susceptible to COVID-19.

In the crossfit community, people were quick to adapt to technology like zoom and google meet to offer workouts and support. My gym, Crossfit Oregon City, let members take equipment home to use while the shelter in place was in effect.

After an adjustment period, we figured out how to do online workouts and to meet with our friends to talk and exercise. It allowed us to have structure in our lives and to keep motivated in keeping fit.

I know for me and my friends it was crucial in keeping our morale high and made the shut down somewhat more bearable.

Right now, we are still in shut down. I know many lessons will come out of this experience that will emphasize the importance of all the things we've talked about in this book. I think if you need any more convincing about how important the elements of connecting are, the pandemic has supplied it.

I hope you are weathering the storm. And I hope you are moving toward fitness.

References

Frankl, V.E. (2006): *Man's Search for Meaning.* Beacon Press.

Glassman, G. (2018): *Level 1 Training Guide 2nd Ed.* Crossfit Inc.

Gundry, S.R., MD (2017): *The Longevity Paradox.* Mercy Book, NY.

Hanh, T.N. (2015): *The Heart of Buddha's Teaching.* United Buddhist Church.

Singh, K.D. (2014): *The Grace in Aging.* Wisdom Publications, Ma.

About the Author

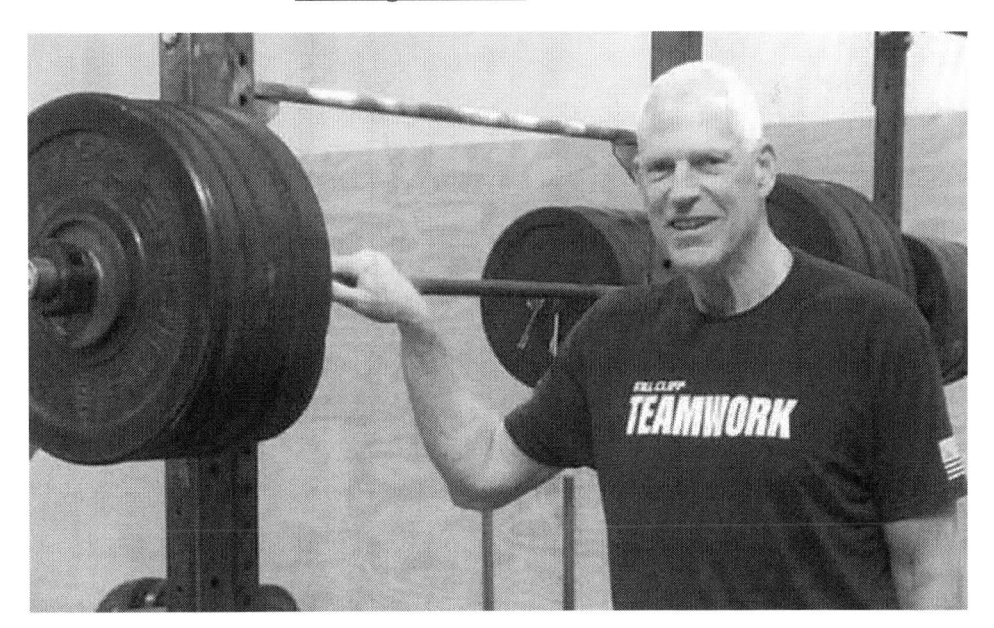

Todd Weber PhD lives in Oregon City, OR with his rescue Catahoula leopard dog, Flash, and his cat, Sammie. He is a former higher education administrator and professor. He currently writes and consults occasionally. Dr. Weber is co-author of the best selling *Drop the Rock* with Bill P. He can be reached at drtoddw@comcast.net

Made in the USA
Columbia, SC
13 July 2020